DR. CHRIS HANNES

Caring for the Horse's Teeth and Mouth

Solving Dental Problems and Improving Health, Comfort, and Performance

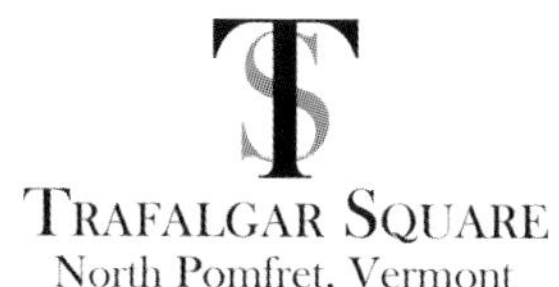

TRAFALGAR SQUARE
North Pomfret, Vermont

First published in the United States of America in 2009 by
Trafalgar Square Books
North Pomfret, Vermont 05053

Printed in China

Originally published in the Dutch language as *Gebitsverzorging bij Paarden* by
Forte Uitgevers bv, Beukenlaan 20, 3741 BP Baarn, The Netherlands

Disclaimer of Liability

The author and publisher shall have neither liability nor responsibility to any person or entity with respect to any loss or damage caused or alleged to be caused directly or indirectly by the information contained in this book. While the book is as accurate as the author can make it, there may be errors, omissions, and inaccuracies.

Library of Congress Cataloging-in-Publication Data

Hannes, Chris.
[Gebitsverzorging bij paarden. English]
Caring for the horse's teeth and mouth : solving dental problems and improving health, comfort, and performance / Chris Hannes.
p. cm.
Includes index.
ISBN 978-1-57076-412-7
1. Equine dentistry. 2. Horses--Diseases. I. Title.
SF959.M66H3613 2009
636.1'089763--dc22
2009002357

Book design: Het vlakke land, Rotterdam
Front cover photos: Big photo, Arnd Bronkhorst, Garderen; small photos, Jolanda Scheepen, Esbeek
Back cover illustration: Nicola Gies
All interior photos are by Chris Hannes *except*: Dr. Bernard Boussauw, veterinary practice De Bosdreef (p.103 *top left*, p.128 *top*); Prof. Paddy Dixon, BEVA and the University of Edinburgh, (p. 1, p. 13 *top left and bottom*, p. 35, p. 68 *bottom right*—from *Equine Dentistry*, Gordon J. Baker and Jack Easley, 2005, Elsevier Saunders—p. 78 *top left*); Dr. Jack Easley, AAEP and the proceedings from the 2006 AAEP Focus on
Dentistry meeting, (p. 82 *top left and top right*); Prof. Dr. Horst Keller (p. 2); Jolanda Scheepen (p. 34, p. 90, p. 93 *top right and bottom left*, p. 98, p. 99, p. 100 *top left*, p. 101, p. 104, p.113); Dr. Marco Van Schie, Lingehoeve Diergeneeskunde (p. 55 *bottom*, p. 78 *top right*, p. 102, p. 103 *top right*); Dr. Lieven Vlaminck, fac. Dierengeneeskunde, University of Gent (p. 43 *top right*, p. 45, p. 67 *bottom right*, p. 80, p. 81, p. 83 *top left and top right*)
Illustrations: Nicola Gies, www.gimoconsultancy.com

The publishers have done their utmost to reach the rightful claimants to the illustrations and photographs. Those who could not be reached in spite of our efforts are requested to make themselves known to the publishers.

10 9 8 7 6 5 4 3 2 1

Contents

Foreword

During the last 10 years, horse dentistry has shown an enormous amount of progress, and this trend is set to continue in the coming years. It is becoming more and more clear just how important the horse's mouth is and, more specifically, the set of the teeth: as a chewing "machine" for efficient processing of food and because of the taxing demands made on this area when the horse is ridden.

This book unravels the secrets and makes short shrift of the myths surrounding dental care for those riders—whether recreational or professional—who have questions, such as: How are the teeth constructed? Why does my horse form wads or balls of hay when he eats? What do the teeth have to do with difficulties riding "on the bit"? What are wolf teeth? What are the benefits of dental care and who should treat the teeth—a dental technician or a veterinarian?

These questions and many more have been addressed and the answers are put clearly into words by an equine veterinarian who has a scientific vision and a passion for horses and their dental concerns. I am sure that you, too, will come to the conclusion that a healthy set of teeth forms the basis of a healthy horse, and that prevention, as always, is better than a cure.

Dr. Lieven Vlaminck
Department of Surgery & Anesthesia for Domestic Animals
Faculty of Veterinary Medicine—University of Ghent, Belgium

Acknowledgments

With thanks to Lieven Vlaminck for a great amount of advice and support and Nicola Gies for the beautiful illustrations. Thanks to Bernard Boussauw, Paddy Dixon, Jack Easley, Horst Keller, Marco Van Schie, and Lieven Vlaminck for the use of their visual material; to Anneke Hallebeek and Paul de Vries for their advice; and to Gertrud Jetten, without whom this book would not have been published.

Introduction

"Don't look a gift horse in the mouth."

This expression definitely doesn't always hold true when you buy a horse or already have one. Indeed, many horses can have early-stage, and even advanced-stage, dental concerns without there being clear symptoms apparent. Horses such as these often suffer in silence.

Teeth disorders can upset nutritional needs, which can then lead to health issues, such as colic, weight loss, diarrhea, and loss of condition. Tooth problems often cause horses to "lean on the bit" and no horse with pain in its mouth can perform its very best.

These days, many horse owners know that dental care for horses exists and is necessary, but most don't have a realistic picture of the horse's mouth and the construction of the teeth. Yet, in equestrian sport, communication with the horse occurs via its mouth. A bad steering wheel in a beautiful car makes it extremely difficult to drive—and the same goes for the horse. What is even worse, in order to escape pain in its mouth, the horse will often react badly to the rider's well-meant rein aids and thus make real riding pleasure impossible.

The aim of this book is to bring insight to horse owners concerning the construction and the workings of a normal set of equine teeth. After all, knowledge is the fount of all wisdom. I begin by showing the normal construction of the mouth and teeth, and then various disorders and their consequences for well-being, feeding, and performance are discussed. I also, explain what is learned from a thorough dental examination and demonstrate how various disorders can be remedied.

The only way to know if your horse has dental problems is for you to have a thorough dental examination carried out by a professional veterinarian or dental technician every year. If necessary, he or she can begin treatment: the ultimate aim of the veterinarian or dental technician is that very same as yours—to have a healthy horse that can perform well.

CHAPTER 1

The History of Equine Dentistry

The first type of horse in existence—the Hyracotherium—lived 55 million years ago in South and Central America. The ancestor of today's horse was then about the size of a dog and mainly fed on soft leaves from the abundance of shrubs present. At that time, this precursor of the horse still had teeth with a short crown—just as humans do. The horse of that period could successfully survive because its teeth were barely worn down by the soft food.

Due to great changes in climate, the vegetation in America changed into vast grasslands of hard pampas grass with low energy yields. The horse also became bigger, so gradually, its energy requirements increased. In order to still take in enough food for energy, the horse needed to graze and chew its food for 18 hours a day. In the following evolutionary phase, due to wear on the teeth, the horse developed a set of teeth with a bigger grinding surface and long "reserve" crowns deep into the socket (see p. 6); these teeth were worn down by the chewing of hard vegetation but at the same rate were continually replaced by new tooth from the socket so that the visible crown stayed the same size in the mouth. After 25 to 30 years, the teeth were completely used up.

It appears from cave drawings in Spain and France that the first contact between humans and horses was around 15,000 BC. At that time,

Below left:
The Hyracotherium, the ancestor of the modern horse, was the size of a dog and lived on a diet of soft leaves. Due to minimal wear, its teeth had short crowns, like ours.

Below right:
The first indication of domestication of horses dates from 4000 BC. Horse skulls from this period were found near the Black Sea: wear and tear on the first molars caused by a bit in the mouth can be seen clearly on the X-ray.

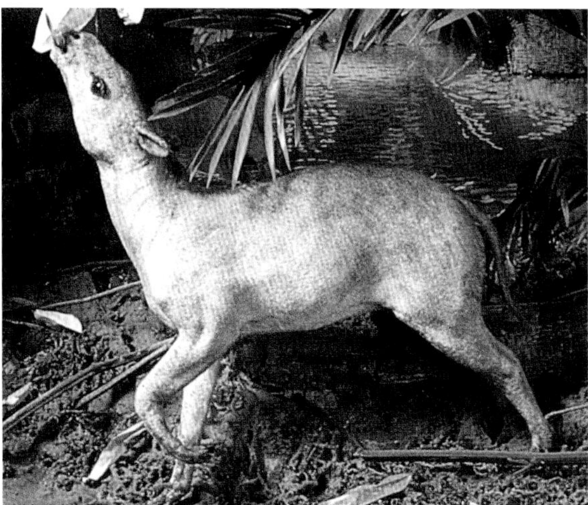

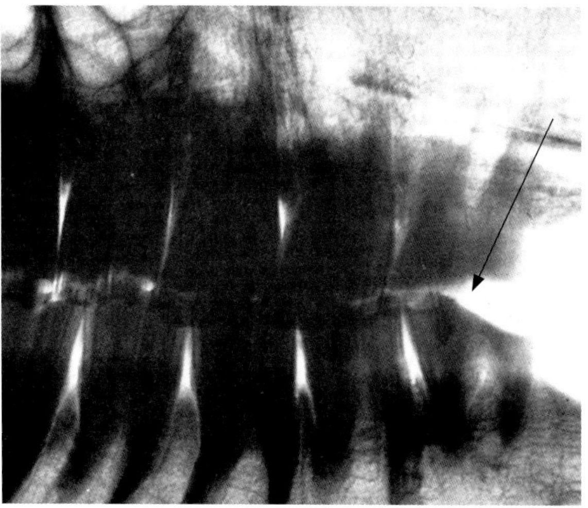

the horse was a source of food for humankind. The cave drawings show images of horses stuck with spears. The first proof that man made use of the horse dates from 4000 BC. In the Black Sea area, the skull of a horse was found from this period that clearly had abrasions of the first molars caused from the use of a bit.

Documentation of horse teeth dates back as early as the ancient Greeks (Xenophon, Aristotle), and the most important aspect of which referred to determining the age of the horse by the "replacement" of the incisors. Even at that time, the age of a horse was relevant for its market value. The wearing down of the incisors was described in the Roman period and permitted the age of a horse to be determined up to the age of 10 years. This information was handed down and taken for granted for more than 10 centuries.

In 1770, in Lyon in France, at the school of veterinary sciences, there was mention of the cutting of the milk teeth and their replacement by permanent teeth. For the first time in many ages, people gained new insights into the teeth of horses by studying the heads of cadavers. Later in 1885, in Alfort, a substantial book was published about the build of the horse, which also fully described the set of teeth of a horse and the determining of age.

At the end of the 19th century, a book was published in England about dental care for horses. This was a project in collaboration between a veterinarian and a dental specialist (note, some people are still calling this a new profession today!). Several firms began making instruments for treatment of horse's teeth. Hand floats designed at that time are still excellent instruments for use in treatment today.

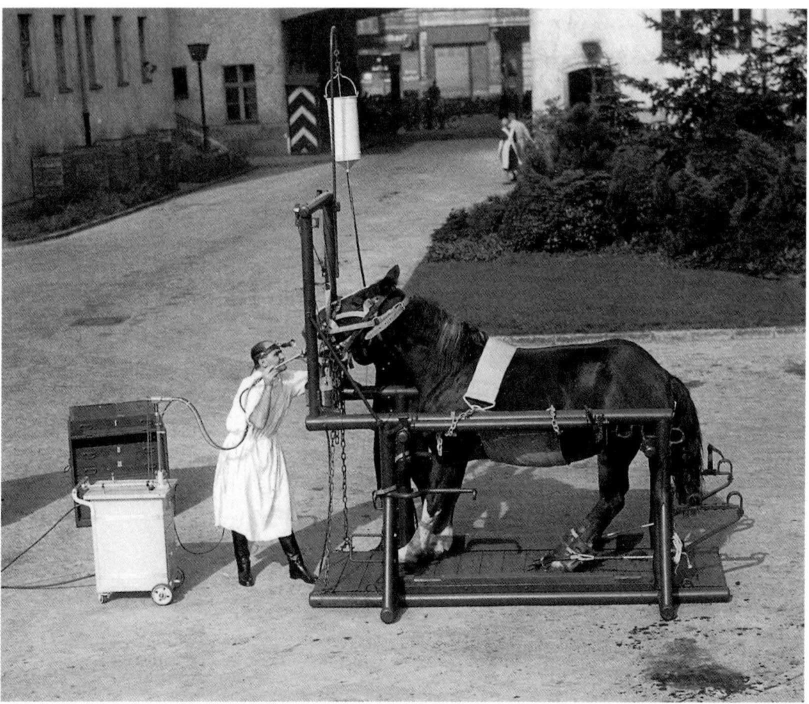

Dental care in Germany around 1940.

In 1904, the first course in equine dentistry was offered at the Detroit Veterinary College. As a means of transport and as a source of power for industry, the horse was extremely important. This is the likely explanation for the growing interest in equine dentistry in the 19th and at the beginning of the 20th century.

After the Second World War, this interest nearly completely disappeared: companies that made the dental instruments were converted to other uses, and interest in horses radically declined due to new forms of transport and the growth of mechanization.

In the 1980s, we witnessed—once again—a return of dental care, despite the fact that it was considered pointless by many horse owners. Nevertheless, from that time, there has been an enormous increase in scientific research on horse's teeth in universities worldwide. Thus, the advantages of caring for the horse's teeth has now been scientifically proved and new treatment protocol developed based on this research.

The array of instruments has expanded enormously in the last twenty years and this has lead to more possibilities for treatment. As well as the existing hand floats, all kinds of electrical floats have been developed. Better dental speculums, portable light sources and such have now made it possible to carry out a thorough examination of the mouth in an animal-friendly manner. The use of anaesthesia for horses has now made the treatment quicker and more efficient.

Within the coming 10 years, every horse owner will consider annual dental treatment as something that goes without saying—just as the bimonthly visit from the farrier already is.

CHAPTER 2

The Anatomy of a Set of Teeth

The set of teeth of a horse consists of 12 incisors and 24 molars; male animals also have four stallion or gelding teeth (the canines). Sometimes, horses may also have two wolf teeth just in front of the molars in the upper jaw; and, there may also be two wolf teeth found in the lower jaw.

There is a very big difference between horse teeth and human teeth. Horse teeth are of the hypsodont type, which have a very long crown that, in a young horse, goes very deeply under the gums into the socket to a relatively short root. The crown is divided into the visible crown (the part you see in the mouth) and the reserve crown (the part of the crown that is still in the socket). Horses need to grind their rough, fibrous rations sufficiently finely with their molars in order to produce a good enzymatic and bacterial digestion in the stomach and the intestines. (The average length of fiber found in a horse's manure is 4 mm). The teeth are

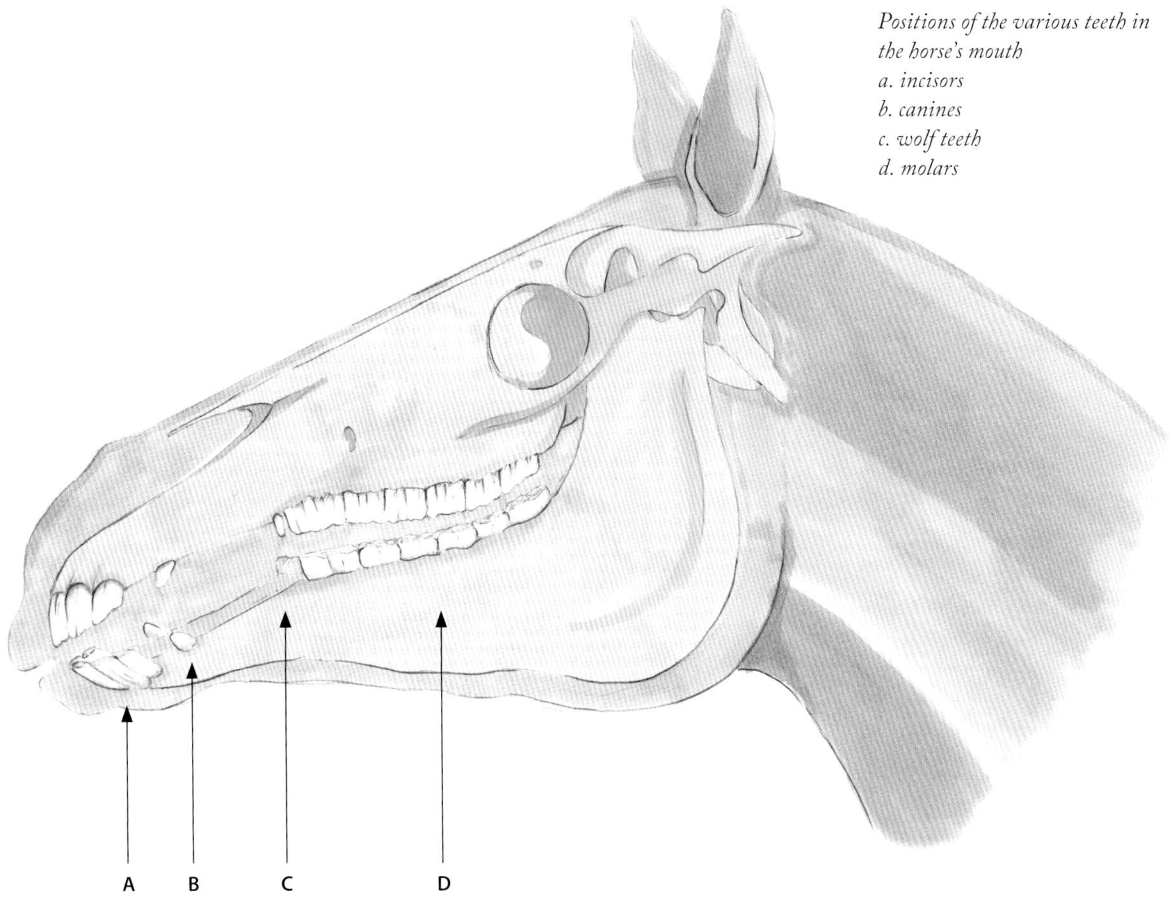

Positions of the various teeth in the horse's mouth
a. incisors
b. canines
c. wolf teeth
d. molars

The horse has hypsodont teeth: a short visible crown with a long "reserve" crown invisible down in the tooth socket and a short root. Humans have brachydont teeth: a relatively short crown, all visible, and a longer root.

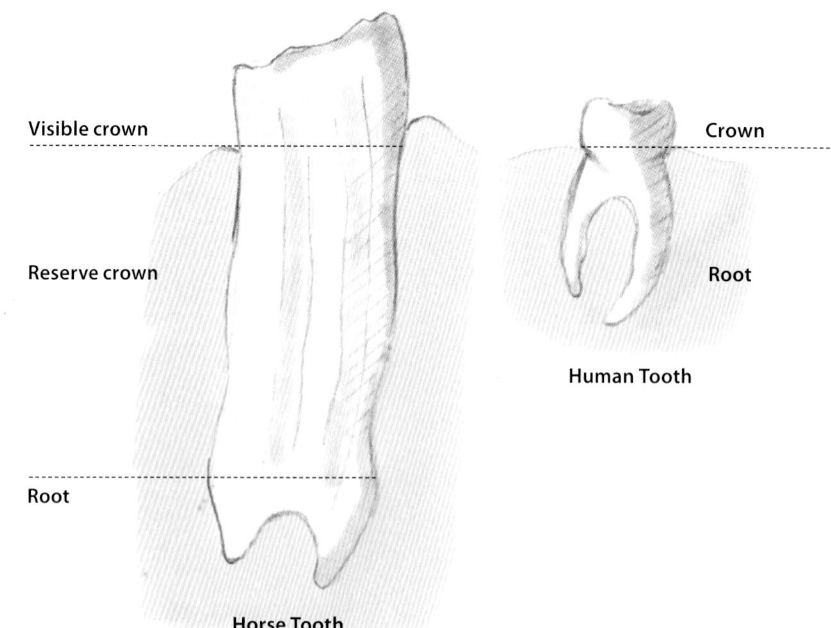

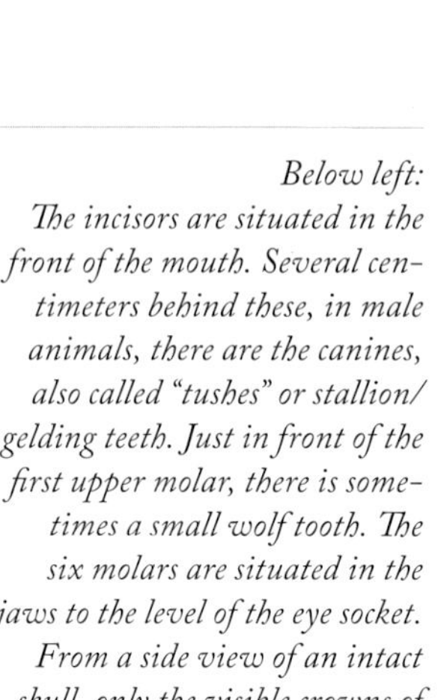

Below left:
The incisors are situated in the front of the mouth. Several centimeters behind these, in male animals, there are the canines, also called "tushes" or stallion/gelding teeth. Just in front of the first upper molar, there is sometimes a small wolf tooth. The six molars are situated in the jaws to the level of the eye socket. From a side view of an intact skull, only the visible crowns of the teeth can be seen.

Below right:
On the left of the picture is the lower jaw and on the right, the upper jaw of an adult horse. Each arcade contains six adjacent teeth. The incisor arc has six incisors. Each jaw, in male animals, has two canines situated behind the incisors. This upper jaw has two wolf teeth just in front of the first molars.

worn down every year by about 2 or 3mm because of the rough fibrous structure of forage.

This wearing down is compensated for by the tooth continually emerging further from the socket—this is called the "eruption" of the teeth. In this way, the part of the tooth above the gums—the visible crown—always remains the same. Human teeth are of the brachydont type, which mean that once the permanent teeth of humans have appeared in the mouth, the tooth has finished growing. The crown is much shorter and ends at the gum where it becomes the root. The crowns present in our mouths must be able to serve us for the rest of our lives. We do not need "horse teeth" because we have a diet of soft food.

In order to avoid misunderstanding, a form of the Triadan system is used to denote specific teeth. Triadan numbering is used worldwide in

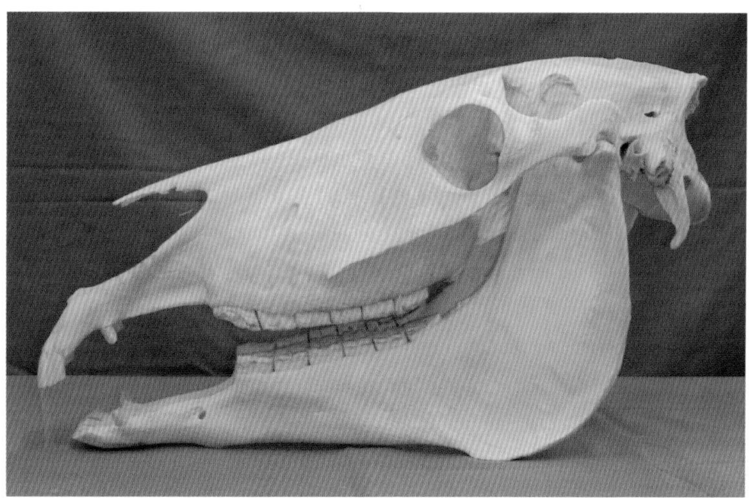

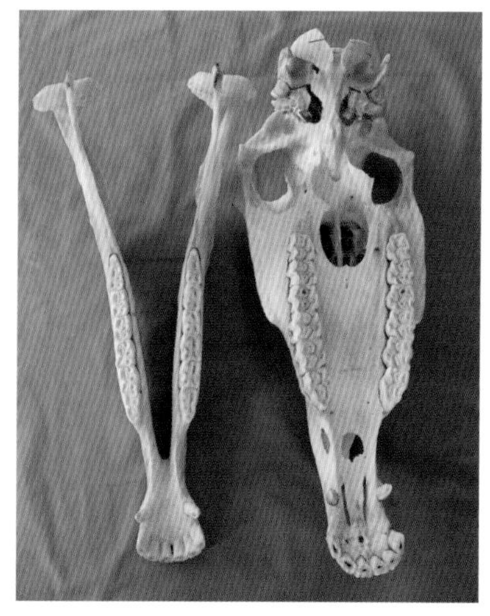

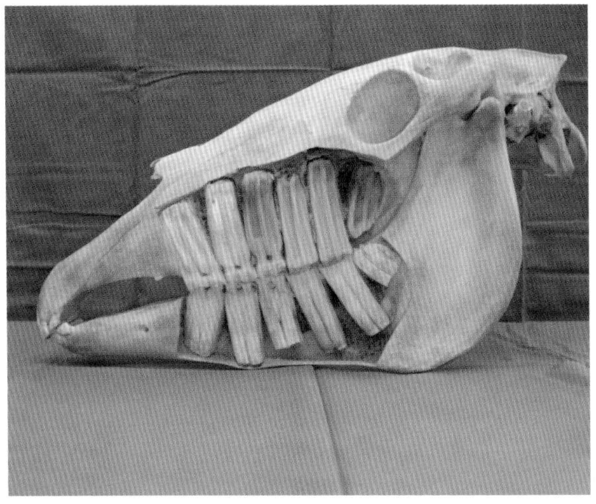

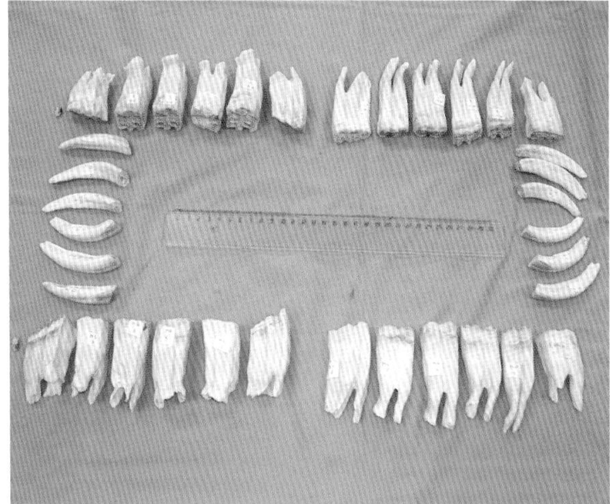

Top left:
Just how long a tooth of a young horse is can only be clearly seen when a skull has been opened up. The "reserve" crown is buried in the tooth's socket. In a young adult, there is still no obvious root present. This is the skull of a 2-year-old.

Top right:
The full set of teeth of an adult mare. No canines are present. At the left are the teeth of the upper jaw, at the right, the teeth of the lower jaw. The molars can be seen horizontally, the incisors vertically. On the far left of the upper set, two small wolf teeth can be seen.

human dentistry. As horses have more teeth than humans, the Triadan system has been adapted but it remains, in principle, the same. This system consists of three numbers and will be used in this book to indicate the tooth denoted.

The first figure denotes which half of the jaw is indicated. The right upper jaw is designated as number 1; the left upper jaw as number 2; the left lower jaw as number 3, and the right lower jaw as number 4. Please note that when stating "left," we mean left from the horse's viewpoint: thus not left as you are standing in front of and facing your horse.

The two numbers that follow thus indicate the specific tooth and in which part of the jaw it is situated. The incisors go from the center to the outside from .01 to .03. If the stallion or gelding tooth is present, it is called .04. Any possible wolf teeth are designated by the number .05. The first to the last molars then receive the numbers .06 to .11. So if we are talking about tooth 310, we are talking about the last but one molar in the left lower jaw.

The Incisors

The two central milk incisors (.01) emerge soon after birth, the next pair—the lateral incisors (.02)—after about 4 to 6 weeks, and the two farthest back—the corner incisors, (.03)—after about 6 to 9 months. The milk incisors are whiter and smaller and have a more clearly defined neck (division between crown and root) and narrower roots than the permanent incisors. The permanent incisors push out the milk incisors from behind and underneath, the roots of which waste away causing the milk teeth to fall out and the permanent incisors to appear. With the central incisors (.01) this happens at the age of 3 years, the lateral ones (.02) at 4 years, and the corner incisors (.03) at 5 years old. These are immutable facts thus they can be soundly used to determine the age of a young horse.

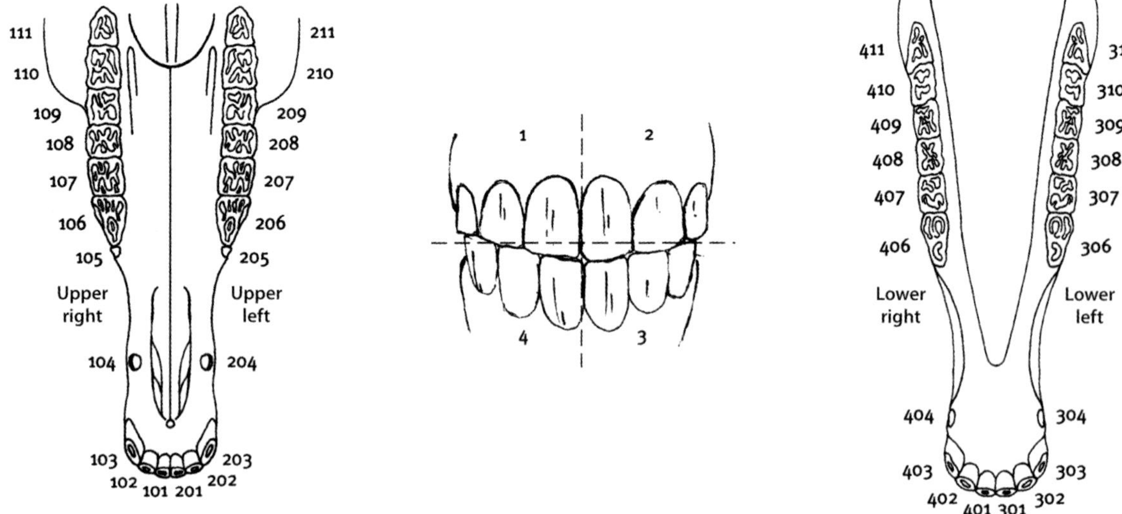

The Triadan system. The set of teeth of a horse is divided into four quadrants. In each quadrant the teeth are designated a number from 1 to 11. Tooth 306 is, thus, the first molar lower left.

On its grinding surface or "table," the incisor has a depression or enamel cup called the "mark." The mark is, in the beginning, about 10mm deep. As the incisor wears down, the mark gradually becomes shallower and finally disappears. On the lip side of the tooth, the dental star appears on the table as the horse gets older. This is actually the top of the root canal, which gradually gets filled up with dentine. Initially the dental star looks like a line parallel with the lip and then, as the horse gets older, the dental star shifts toward the middle of the table and it becomes rounder. The dental star often has a yellow-to-brownish tint due to the effect of staining from grass pigment. As the horse ages, a white fleck appears in the center of the dental star. The mark in the crown and the dental star are also used to determine age. The rapidity of the wearing down is indeed determined by, among other things, the makeup of the diet (little or much roughage) and the differences in tooth composition and sometimes by external factors such as crib biting. Formerly, this knowledge was also regularly used to falsify the age of a horse by filing away the surface of the incisor.

Galvayne's groove is a vertical groove on the lip side of the upper corner incisors. This groove originates at the edge of the gum and becomes longer with age until the groove reaches the nipping surface. Formerly Galvayne's groove was also used to determine age. However, this groove is absent in 50 percent of horses.

Horses often develop a hook on the back edge of the nipping surface of the upper corner incisor called the échancrure or notch. It used to be thought that these horses were 7 to 13 years old: this parameter is, however, totally untrustworthy as a method of determining the age of a horse.

The gap between the incisors and the first molar is called the interdental space or bar. The bit rests in this place. The thin soft tissue of the

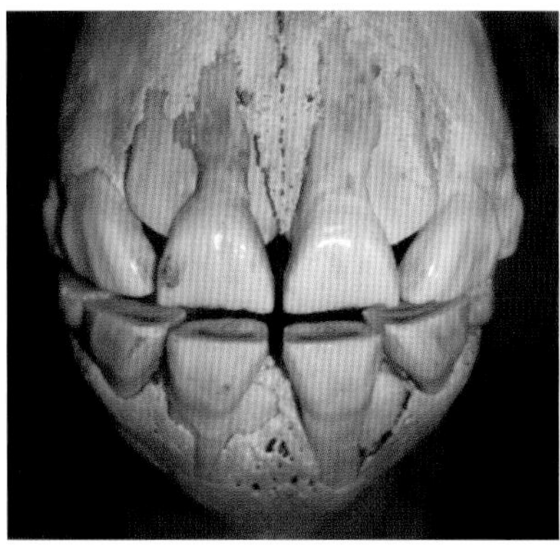

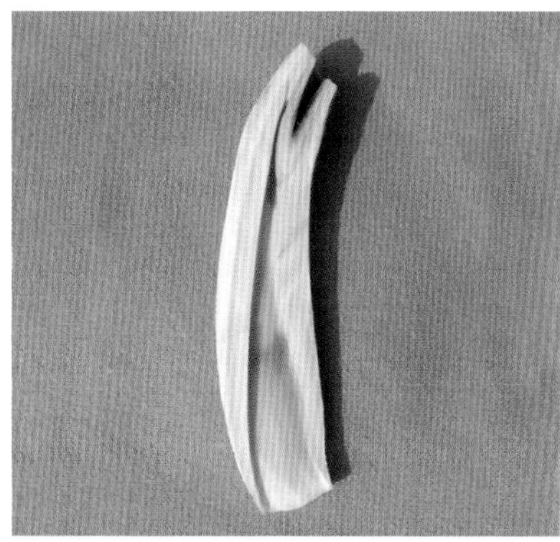

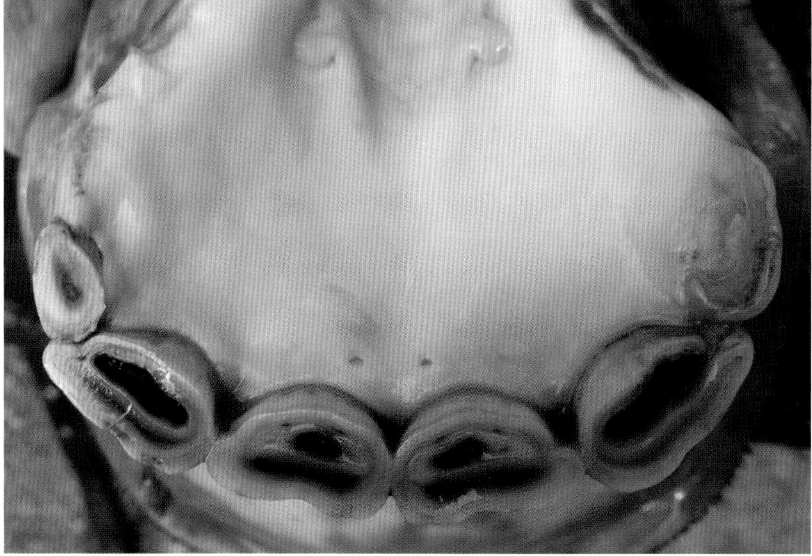

Top left:
When the central permanent incisors erupt they push out the roots of the central milk incisors so in the end, they fall out into the mouth and the horse's teeth have been replaced. This is a skull of a 2½ year old horse: the replacement of the central incisors is nearly complete.

Top right:
A lengthwise cross section of a permanent incisor of a young adult horse. The mark or enamel cup in the crown can be clearly seen in the cross section: it is nearly 1 cm deep. The root canal narrows towards the incisor table. As the wearing-down process of the incisors progresses, the enamel cup and the top of the root canal gradually gets filled up with dentine. If this wasn't the case, the root canal would be opened up by the wearing-down process and, eventually, this would lead to the loss of the incisor. The filled root canal can later be seen on the lip side of the table in the form of the dental star. The passage of the root canal makes it clear why the dental star, in a young horse, is in the front of the tooth and in an old horse situated centrally on the table.

Below:
The lower incisors of a 4½-year-old horse. At the far left, a milk incisor can still be seen. On the far right, the permanent third incisor is erupting from the gums. On the central permanent incisors a slight depression can still be seen on the table: the mark or glazed cup. The black line on the lip side is the stripe-shaped dental star. The lateral permanent incisors have even deeper marks and as yet, no dental star. Note also the oval table of the incisors following the line of the incisor arc—a characteristic of young horses.

mouth covers the hard underlying bone. We often see injuries on the bar of the lower jaw in horses that are ridden with a curb bit.

The Canines

The canines, also known as the tushes, stallion, or gelding teeth (.04), are found in male animals a few centimeters behind the last incisor. Sometimes mares have extremely small canines that can be seen or felt under the soft tissue. Originally, this tooth was used by males as a defence weapon but, with the advance of evolution, it has become defunct in the modern horse. These teeth erupt at about 4 1/2 to 5 years old in both the upper and lower jaw. It is usually pointed and quite sharp. Seeing that the lower canine is further forwards than the upper canine, there is no wearing out of the visible crown by grinding. After their eruption in the mouth, these teeth do not continue to emerge from their sockets as do the incisors and molars. During the whole life of the horse, the long reserve crowns of the canines remain buried in their sockets.

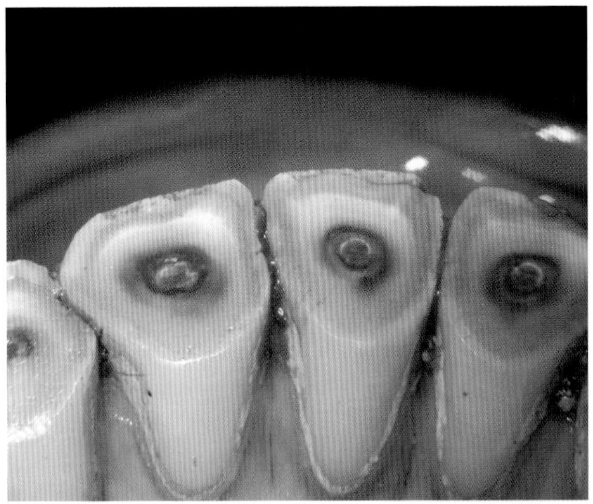

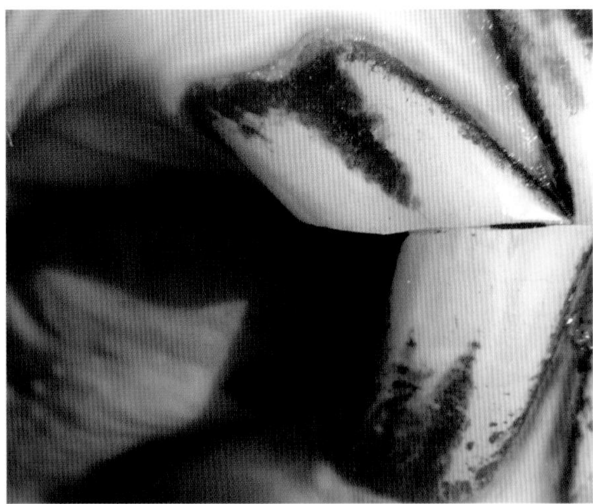

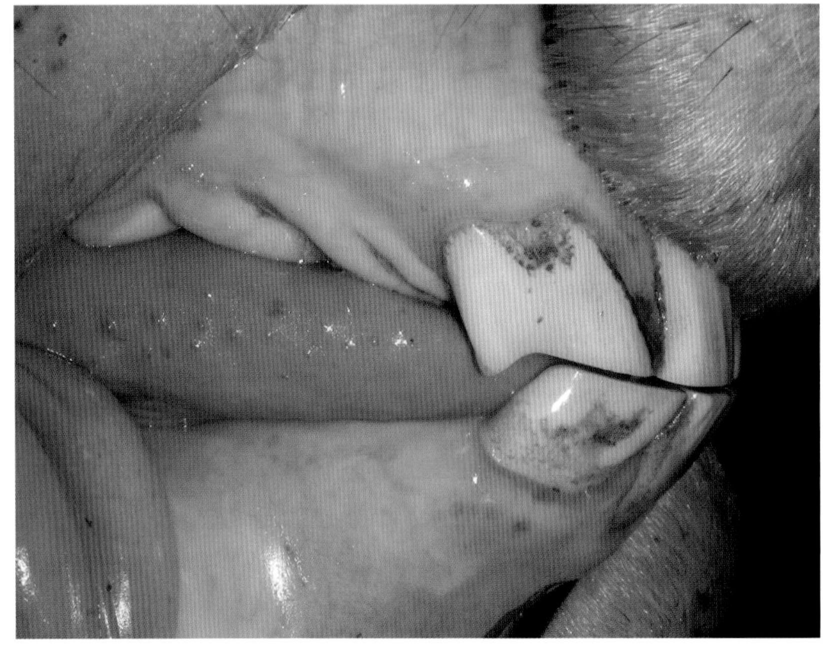

Top left:
The incisors of a 25-year-old horse. The tables of these incisors have become more of a rectangle positioned crossways to the incisor arc, and the marks have completely disappeared. The dental stars are now circular and are situated in the middle of the tables.

Top right:
The groove that gradually appears at the lip side of the corner incisor of the upper jaw is called Galvayne's groove. In former times, this groove was—quite mistakenly—used to determine the age of a horse.

Below:
The hook at the back of the corner incisor in the upper jaw is also known as an échancrure or notch. It used to be thought that this appeared at a certain age and it was incorrectly used to determine the age of a horse.

The Wolf Teeth

Wolf teeth (.05) are usually small teeth of about 1 to 2 cm long, which are situated just in front of the upper molars. The visible crown is mostly only a few millimeters long. Wolf teeth are present in the upper jaw of 20 to 30 percent of horses. Very occasionally, wolf teeth can be seen just in front of the first molar in the lower jaw; they are usually much smaller than the wolf teeth in the upper jaw.

Wolf teeth appear in the mouth between 8 months and 1 1/2 years. Long ago in the evolution of the horse, these teeth formed an extra set and were then much bigger. In the modern horse they are completely redundant.

"Blind" wolf teeth are situated 1 to 2 cm in front of the first molar and

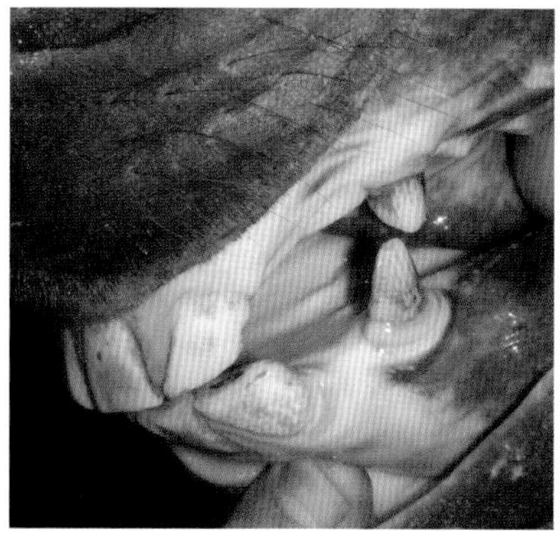

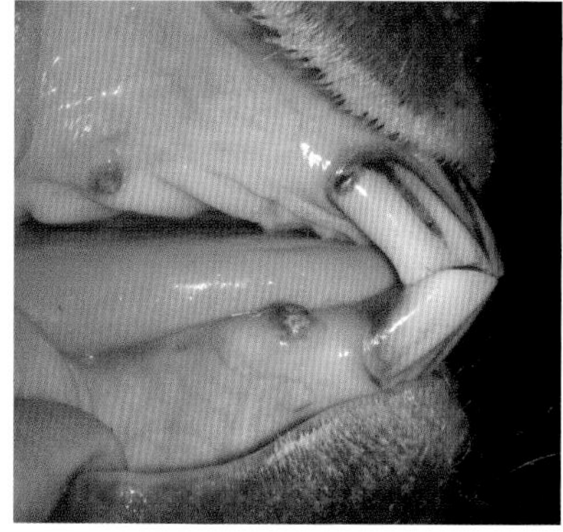

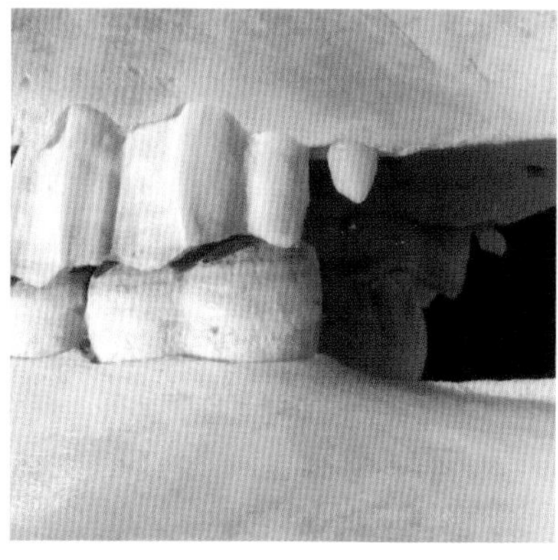

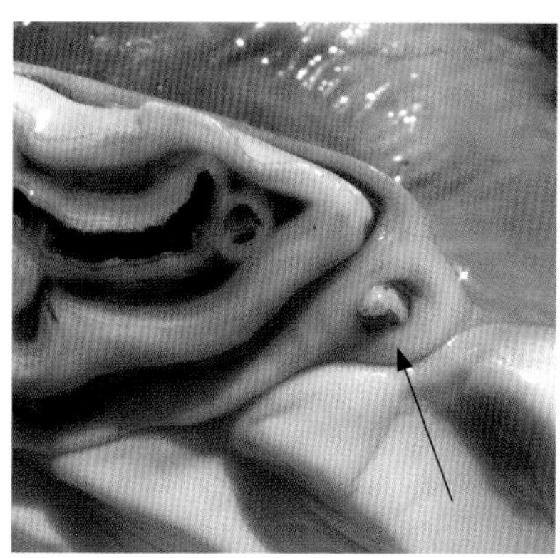

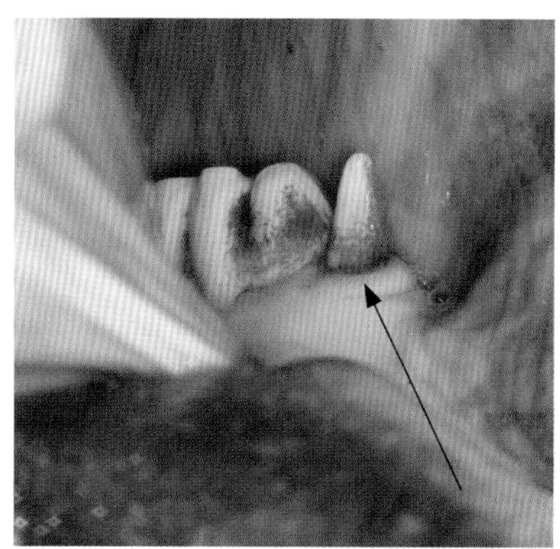

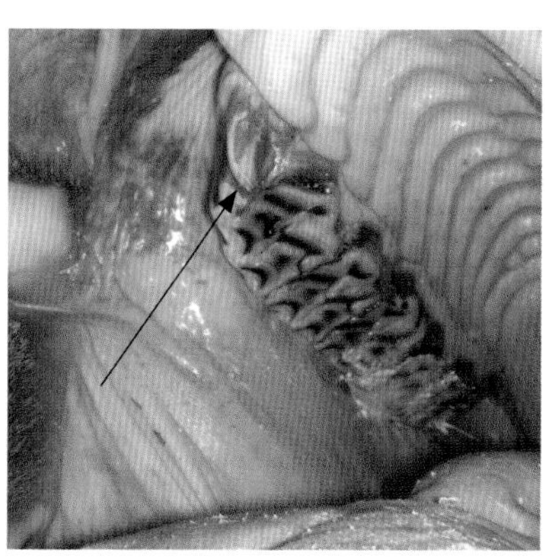

Top left:
In male animals, from the age of 5 years old, canines are present behind the incisors. The upper canines are further back than the lower canines: the two sets do not touch. Once upon a time, these teeth were used as a defensive weapon but in today's horse, these teeth are defunct.

Top right:
Some adult mares have tiny canines. They are just appearing through the gums in this mare.

Middle left:
Small wolf teeth are present just in front of the first molars in 20 to 30 percent of horses.

Middle right:
The table of the first molar of the upper jaw can be seen. In front of it is the tiny pointed crown of the wolf tooth. Note the enormous difference in size between the two.

Below left:
Some horses also have a wolf tooth in front of the first molar in the lower jaw. Thus, sometimes a horse can have four wolf teeth.

Below right:
Sometimes wolf teeth can be extremely big. This wolf tooth was quite a size at 4 cm long.

are mostly implanted slanting toward the front and thus, do not erupt from the soft tissue; they can only be felt as a knob under the skin at the level of the bar.

Wolf teeth can be a reason why some sport horses "lean on the bit" and the ensuing problems. As these teeth no longer have a function in the mouth, they are often removed at the beginning of a sport horse's career.

The Molars

The first three milk molars (.06 to .08) are already present in the first week of the foal's life. These teeth are replaced by the permanent teeth

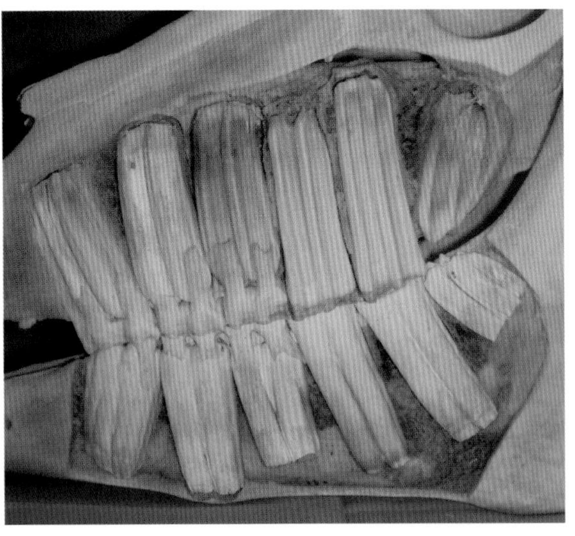

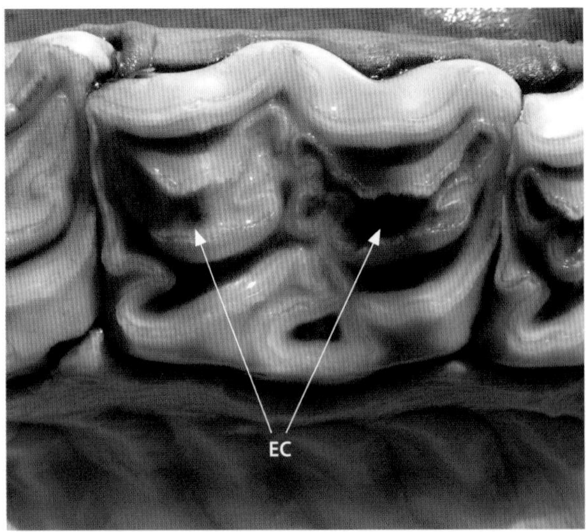

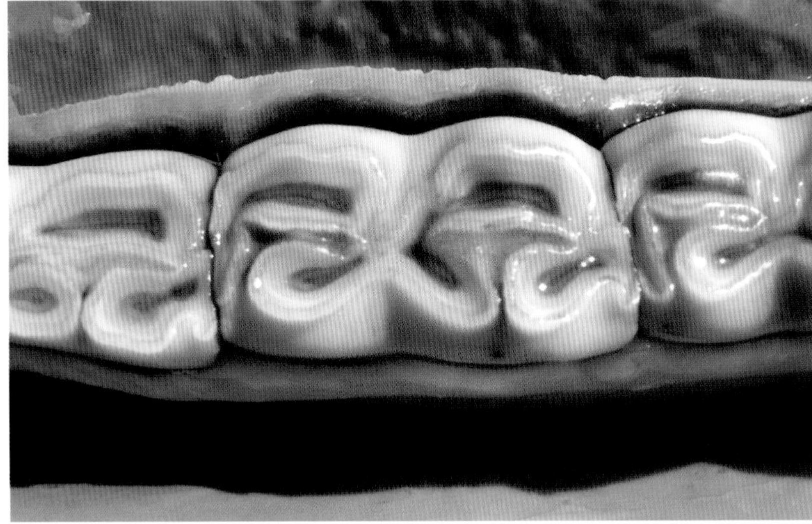

Top left:
The skull of a 2½-year-old horse. Remains of the milk teeth can clearly be seen on the tables of the first three molars. These are eventually pushed out into the mouth as "caps." The last three molars arriving as permanent teeth thus have no caps. Tooth four and tooth five have already erupted into the mouth; tooth six is on the point of doing so. It can be seen that the tables of the arcade of teeth slightly curve up towards the back. The first molar is implanted at an angle towards the back and the last two molars are implanted slanting forward. This construction means that all the teeth are pushed against each other and form a compact whole.

Top right:
In the rectangular-shaped upper molar two enamel cups filled with cementum can be seen in the middle (EC).

Below:
The tables of the lower molars are narrower and have no enamel cups.

at 2½ years (.06), 3 years (.07), and 4 years old (.08). The force of the emerging permanent teeth destroys the roots of the much shorter milk teeth and pushes the remaining parts of the milk teeth into the mouth. These remains of milk teeth—the "caps"– can sometimes be found in the horse's feeding container. These caps are usually thin, rectangular slivers with a few sharp remains of the root on the edge.

The last three molars (.09 to .11) appear only once, that is, they arrive as permanent teeth. These appear in the mouth as a 1-year-old (.09), 2 years old (.10) and 3½ years old (.11). Thus, in an adult horse, the fourth molar (.09) is the oldest tooth in its mouth.

The upper molars have two depressions centrally placed on the grinding surface or table of the crown. As opposed to the incisors, in the beginning these "marks" or enamel cups are not concave but completely filled with cementum and they also reach to just above the root of the tooth. The lower molars do not have enamel cups.

The molars fit beautifully together and form a nearly level surface that

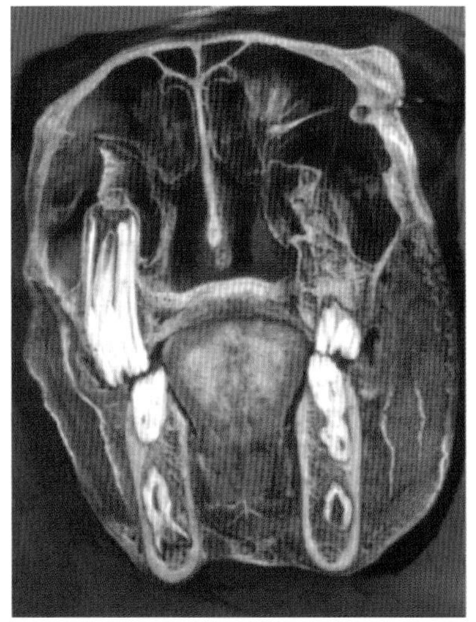

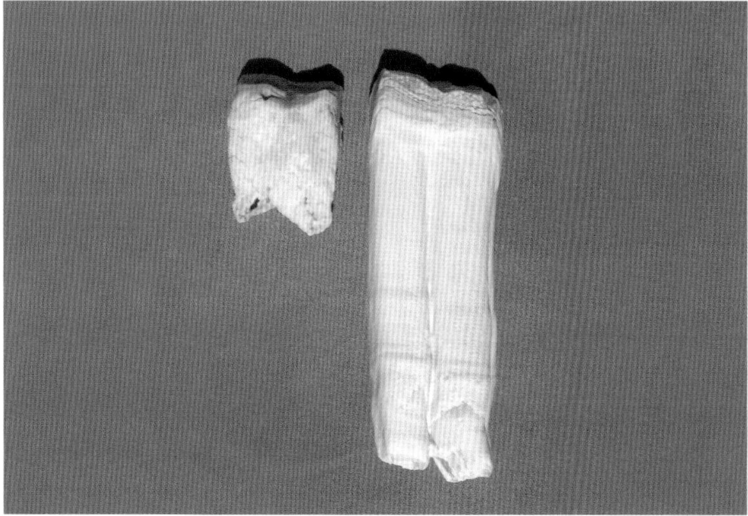

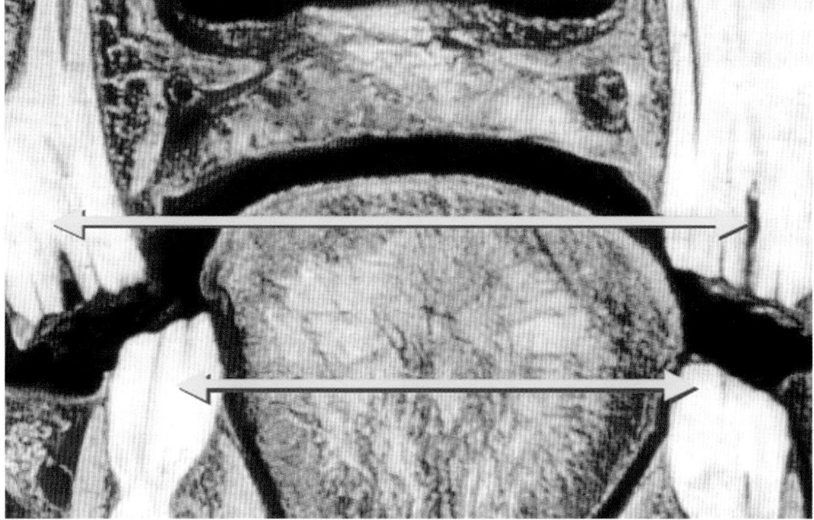

Top left:
A cross section of a horse's head at the level of the fifth molar. At the left in the picture, you can see that the root of the molar, in a young horse, reaches as far as the sinus cavity. An infection of the molar root in a young horse can thus easily lead to an infection of the adjacent sinus.

Above right:
On the right is a molar of a young adult horse; this molar is a good 10 cm long. On the left is a molar that has been extracted from a 28-year-old, the crown of which is only 2 cm long. The rest of the crown has disappeared due to natural wearing down when feeding.

Below:
In this cross section of a horse's head at the level of the molars, the upper molars are not positioned directly on top of the lower molars; the table of the upper molars is wider than that of the lower ones; the tables do not fit together horizontally but are set at an angle of about 15 degrees. Sharp enamel points often develop on the outer edge of the upper molars—these can injure the inside of the cheek.

gradually curves up toward the back of the mouth. This upward curve is known as the "Spee curvature." The root of the first molar is implanted a little forwards and the roots of the last two molars are implanted slightly backward. With this pressure from both ends of the arcade of teeth, the molars remain nicely compact and the six individual teeth act as a single unit.

The table of most of the molars is rectangular. The tables of the upper teeth are much broader than those of the lower teeth; the upper teeth are also spread 30 percent wider than the lower teeth. This means that, when at rest, only half of the grinding surface of the upper teeth is placed above the outside third of the grinding surface of the lower teeth. Additionally, the tables aren't horizontal but slanted outwards at an angle of about 10 to 25 percent. All these factors in the construction of the upper teeth explain why we so often see injuries in the soft tissue of the cheek that are caused by sharp glazed points on the outside of the chewing surface of the upper molars.

On each complete arcade of teeth there are 11 to 13 transverse ridges on the grinding surface. These ridges ensure a multiplication of the chewing surface of the molars and are a normal and useful phenomenon in a horse.

In the young horse, the roots of the last four upper molars reach to just under the bottom of the sinuses. The sinuses are hollow spaces in the forehead of a horse. This proximity can mean that a bacterial infection of these roots could also cause an infection of the sinuses.

A mature molar is up to 10 cm long of which the greater part is to be found in the socket. As mentioned, during the lifetime of the horse, the reserve crown gradually and continually erupts from the socket at a rate of 2 to 3 mm a year. At about 30 to 35 years old, the roots appear at the surface and the rest of the tooth falls out by degrees.

The Skull

The skull is made up of two halves: the lower half consists of only two

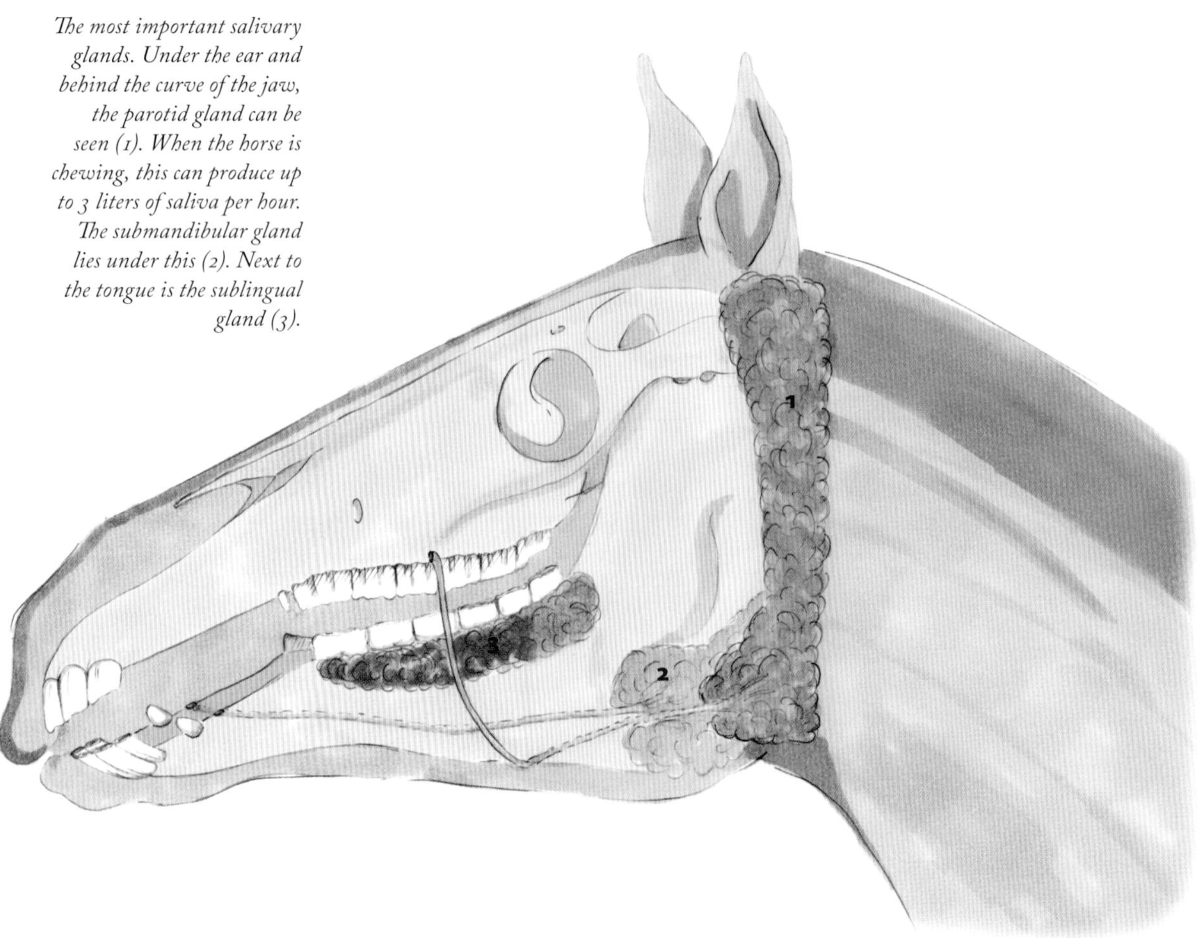

The most important salivary glands. Under the ear and behind the curve of the jaw, the parotid gland can be seen (1). When the horse is chewing, this can produce up to 3 liters of saliva per hour. The submandibular gland lies under this (2). Next to the tongue is the sublingual gland (3).

bones that join together in the front, that is, the branches of the lower jaw or rami mandibulae together form the lower jaw. The upper half consists of a collection of several bone parts including the upper jaw part. The lower jaw can, via the jaw joint, move in three directions in relation to the upper jaw. The horse can move its mouth quite far—up and down and sideways. The forward and backward movement of both jaws, in relation to each other, is limited (6 to 8 mm). With each of these movements it is always the lower jaw which moves in relation to the upper jaw. The outer side of the jaw joint can be felt on the outside of the head just in front of the base of the ear.

The Salivary Glands

On each side of its head the horse has three salivary glands of which the biggest is the parotid gland. This is found behind the jaw and under the ear, and when the horse is chewing, it produces 50 ml of saliva a minute: thus, a production of 3 liters of saliva per hour. The gland discharges into

The horse has enormous muscles for chewing (the masseter); these should be symmetrically developed on both sides of the head.

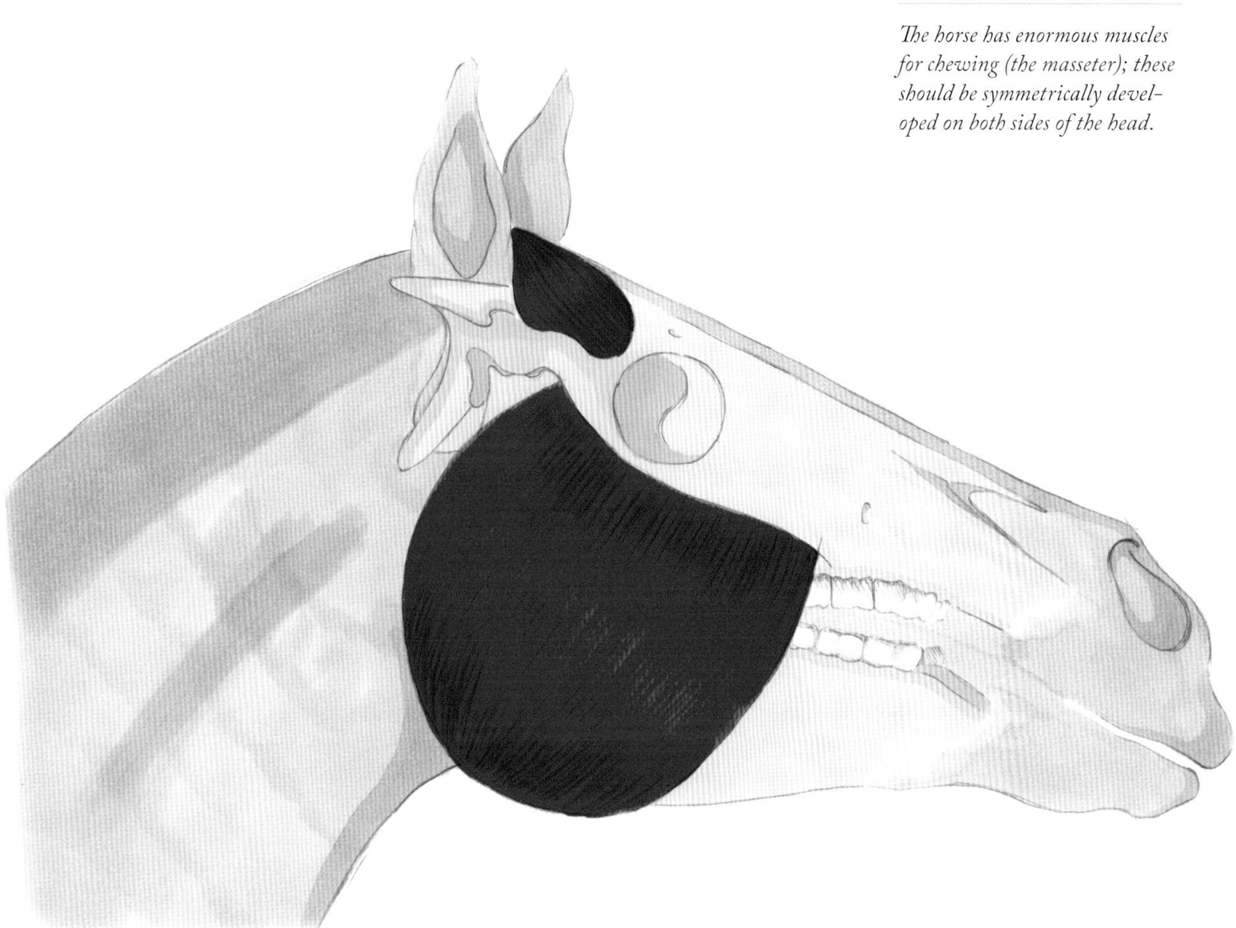

the mouth cavity at the level of the third upper molar via the cheek. The drainage channel of this salivary gland commences along the inside of the lower jaw. At the front of the masseter (the muscle for chewing), the channel goes under the lower jaw through to the outside of the lower jaw where it lies just below the skin. An injury at this spot can cause an opening in the channel; you will then see saliva flow from the wound when the horse is eating.

In the spring, when horses are first put out onto grass, this gland can sometimes swell up a lot. The reason for this is still not known. Fortunately, after a night of rest in its stall with its head in the normal raised position, the swelling usually subsides.

The smaller, submandibular salivary gland is situated behind the lower jaw curve and it discharges into the mouth cavity in the inside at the level of the canines. The sublingual salivary gland under the tongue lies on both sides just under the soft tissue and has several openings into the mouth cavity.

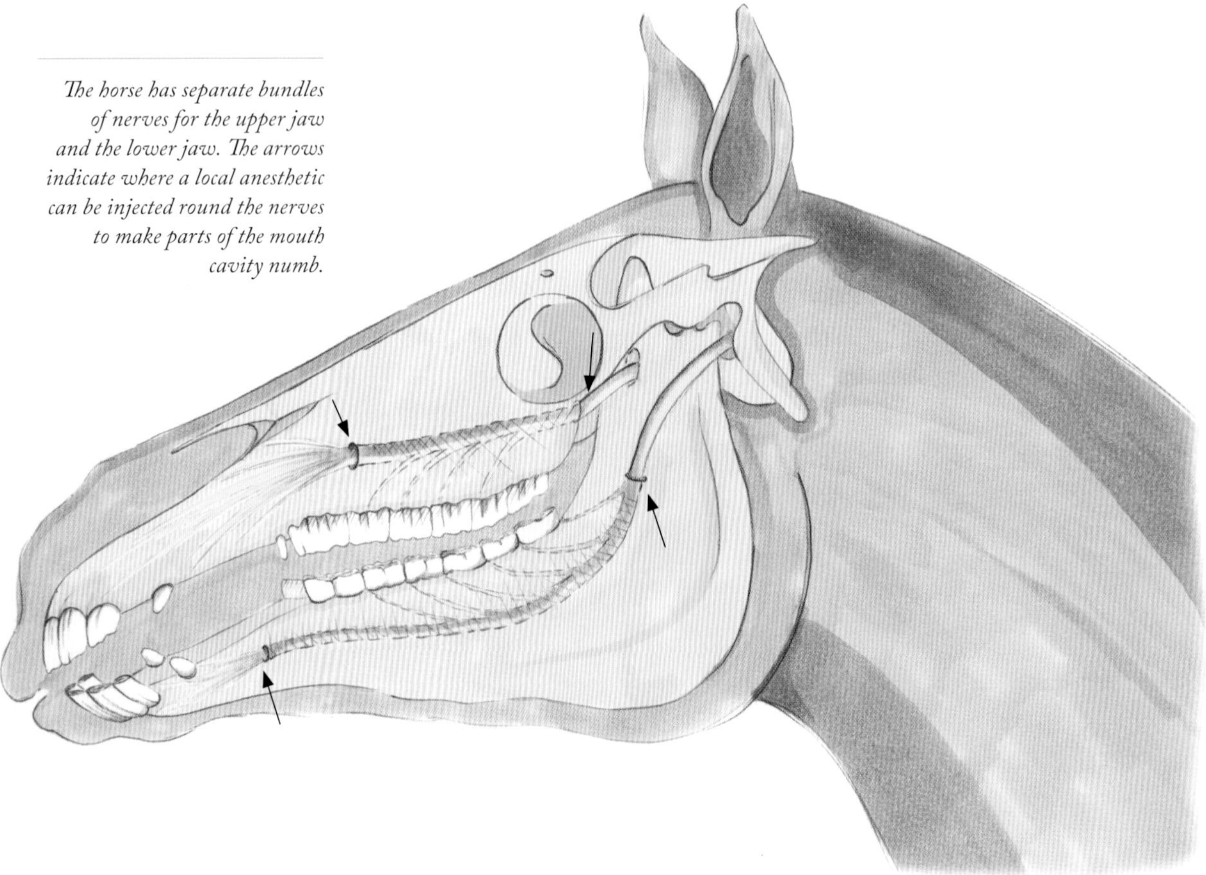

The horse has separate bundles of nerves for the upper jaw and the lower jaw. The arrows indicate where a local anesthetic can be injected round the nerves to make parts of the mouth cavity numb.

The Masseters

Far back in the past, fodder for horses consisted of tough grass and, in times of scarcity, roots and branches. Therefore, the horse needed strong chewing muscles to finely grind all this between its molars. The well-developed masseters can, for a large part, be palpated on both sides of the head and should be nicely symmetrical. The chewing muscles that are most well developed are those needed to close the mouth and those for food grinding. Muscles used for mouth opening are less well developed: indeed, opening the mouth can occur with very little resistance.

The Nerves

It is a frequently heard misconception that the teeth of the horse have no feeling because they don't have nerves. But, it has long been scientifically proved that nerve fibers enter through the root opening into the root canal of the tooth.

The nerves that lead to the teeth arrive as one bundle from the cranial cavity to the outer side of the skull where they divide to form one bundle for the lower jaw and one bundle for the upper jaw.

The nerve bundle for the upper jaw continues along the underside of the eyeball and, at that point, turns back into the bony part of the upper jaw. Within this bone, fine nerve branches divide and lead to the upper molars. At the height of the third molar, the nerve reappears at the surface of the bone and runs under the skin to the lip. This bony opening can be felt on the outside of the skull.

The nerve bundle for the lower jaw continues along the inside of the jaw curve and then disappears into an opening in the bone after which several nerve branches lead to the various lower molars. A few centimeters in front of the first molar, the nerve reappears on the outside of the lower jaw bone where, just below the skin surface, it continues to the lip. This opening, too, can be felt in the lower jaw.

In the places where the nerve burrows into the bone or where it resurfaces, certain parts of the mouth can be made numb by an injection of liquid anesthetic to produce pain-free treatment whenever necessary. Horses can often react violently when the nerve in the opening is pierced by the needle.

Acute toothache from extreme heat or cold as experienced by humans probably does not exist in horses. There are indications that the opening of the root canal by exaggerated filing can be responsible for transitory gnawing pain in the tooth. If a horse breaks a tooth and the root canal is opened, the animal never displays symptoms of toothache (such as "quidding," which is allowing feed to drop from the mouth) or radiant pain in the surrounding jaw bone.

CHAPTER 3

The Composition of the Tooth

The teeth are built up of three elements: dentine, enamel and cementum. Each element has its specific function in the construction of the tooth. Underneath the tooth is the root aperture (molars have more than one) that continues up through the tooth as the root canal.

The Dentine

The major part of the tooth is composed of dentine. This is a cream-colored substance that is much softer than enamel but less fragile. The dentine supports the harder, but more brittle enamel against breakage in the tooth. The unequal hardness of the two substances is the cause of an irregular pattern of wearing down on the table: the enamel wears down more slowly than the dentine and cementum. The enamel stands somewhat higher on the table than the other substances that make up the tooth. This rough and, at the same time, larger grinding surface makes for more efficient chewing.

As opposed to enamel, dentine is continually being produced in an adult tooth. If this was not the case, the top of the root canal would gradually appear on the table surface due to the wearing-down process; this could then cause root canal infection. As the tooth is worn down, new dentine is deposited on the surface of the root canal under the influence of the mechanical pressure. The fact that dentine absorbs grass pigment can clearly be seen from the brown tint of the dental star in the incisors.

The Enamel

Enamel or dental enamel is the hardest substance in the body. In horses, the enamel on the outside of the tooth is for a great part covered by a layer of matt cementum except on the chewing surface. This cementum is often worn off on the front of the incisors by forage so that the shiny aspect of the enamel appears on the surface. The milk teeth of a horse are usually a little whiter because less cementum is present. Although enamel is extremely resistant to friction on the surface of the table, it is

Top:
Here the permanent lower incisors of a 5-year-old horse can be seen. The incisors have, on the outside, a thin layer of cementum that envelops the white enamel underneath (E). Centrally placed on the table is an oval enamel ring (ER) that forms the mark or the enamel cup. The base of the mark is filled with cementum (C), as can be seen on the table of the central incisor (.01). Between the outside layer of enamel and the inside enamel ring there is dentine (D). This brownish, line-like discoloration of the dentine in the central incisor is the dental star (DS). This is the top of the root canal, which is filled with dentine—made clear in the following diagram.

Below left:
The outside of the incisor is made of enamel covered with a layer of cementum. The enamel cup or mark (M) is confined by enamel. The base of this depression is filled with cementum. The remainder of the incisor consists of dentine that envelops the root canal (RC). As the incisor is worn away, the top of the root canal gets filled with dentine to prevent an opening appearing in the root canal; this later becomes visible as the dental star.

Below right:
The same components can be seen here illustrated in outline: D=dentine; E=enamel; C=cementum; M=mark; RC=root canal.

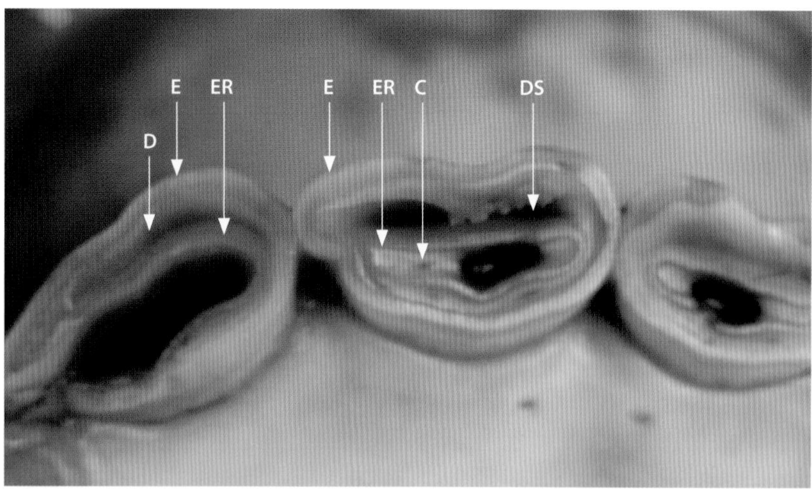

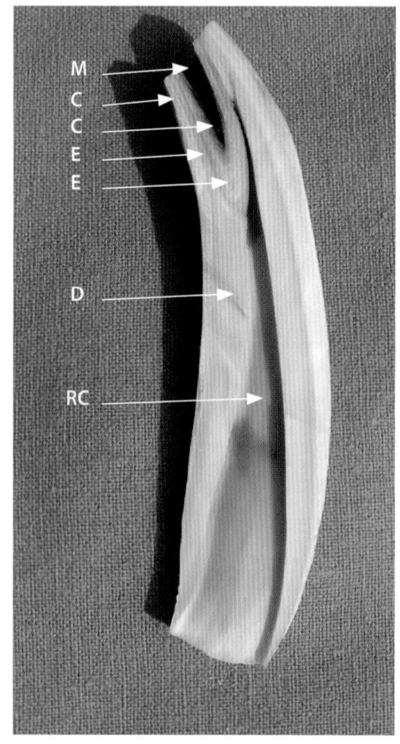

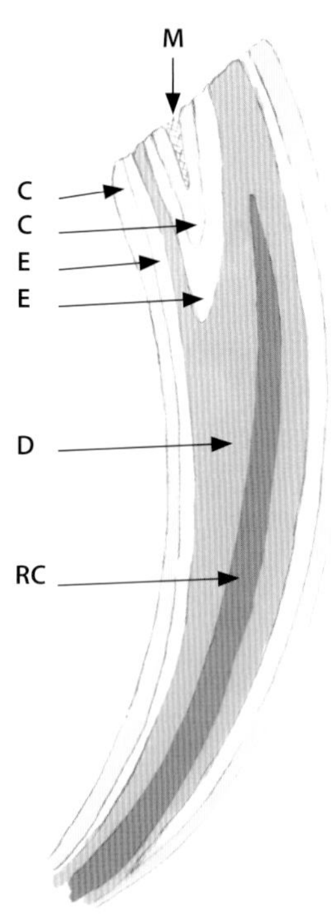

very brittle and it breaks rather easily. It needs to be supported by the other tissues of the tooth.

In the incisor, the enamel surrounds the whole crown just under the cementum and is nearly parallel with the outside of the tooth. The crown depression—or "mark"—is also confined like this. In the molars, the enamel is also on the outside just under the cementum but it is much more undulating. We shall see that this plays a role in the development of the enamel points that can cause a lot of problems for a horse.

The upper molars have, centrally in the tooth, two extra undulated enamel "rings" or indentations that are filled with cementum—the "marks" or enamel cups.

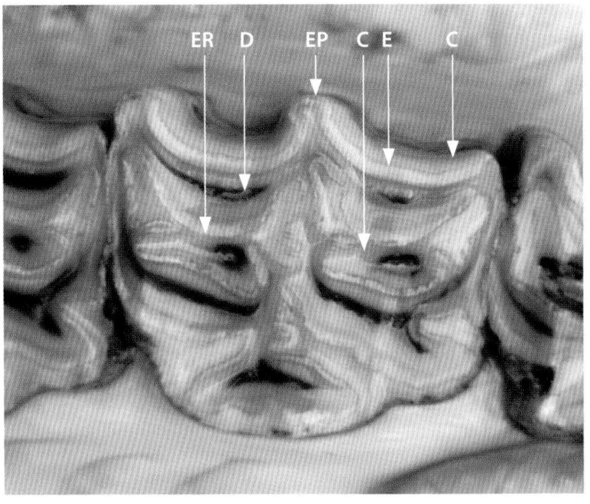

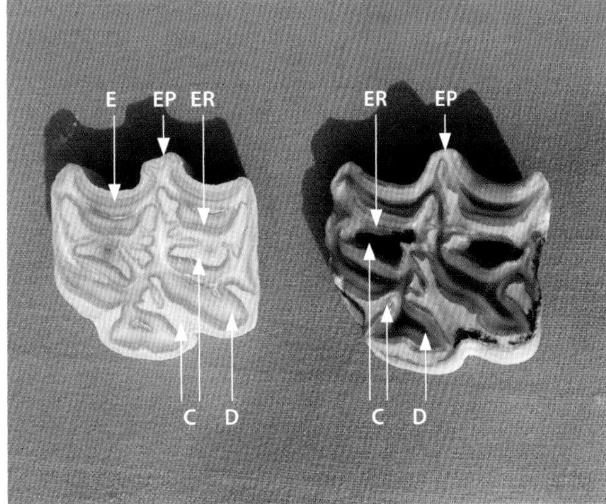

Left:
Here the table of the upper molars can be seen. The shiny white is the rather twisting enamel line (E). At the cheek side of the molar, the enamel line is wavy: the cause of the sharp enamel points (EP). Centrally situated in the molar are the two wavy enamel "rings" (ER)—the enamel cups or marks. The outside of the tooth and the filling of the central enamel ring consist of cementum (C). Between the outer enamel line and the two enamel "rings" there is dentine (D).

Right:
Comparison between an upper molar table and the cross section of an upper molar sliced 1 cm below the table surface. (Left: the cross-section. Right: the complete tooth.) The various components of the teeth can be seen more clearly.

The Cementum

Cementum is a cream-colored, chalky substance that shares characteristics with normal bone tissue. This is the softest element of the tooth. Cementum envelops the whole crown of the tooth on the outside.

Cementum can build up—just as dentine can—in an adult tooth, for example, by trauma or bacterial infection. The tissues that radiate from the cementum of the reserve crown are firmly anchored in the surrounding bone of the socket and thus ensure that the teeth are solidly embedded in the tooth socket.

The Root Canal

Nerve fibers and blood vessels are able to enter the hollow root canal via the root aperture. Incisors and canines have only a single root and root canal. The lower molars have two roots (but the last lower molar has three) and the upper molars have three roots. Depending on their position in the arcade of teeth, the molars have five to seven root canals.

Due to the good supply of blood in the tooth (a good supply of defensive cells) and the possibility of depositing dentine, an opening of the root canal in the mouth of a horse doesn't often result in the loss of a tooth, as would be the case with humans. The possibility of infection is suppressed by defensive cells and the newly deposited dentine seals the root canal again. With aging, the root cavity increasingly reduces in size because of the dentine deposits on the chewing end. When the molars are nearly completely worn down, the root canal is completely filled with dentine and the root canal is thus no longer present.

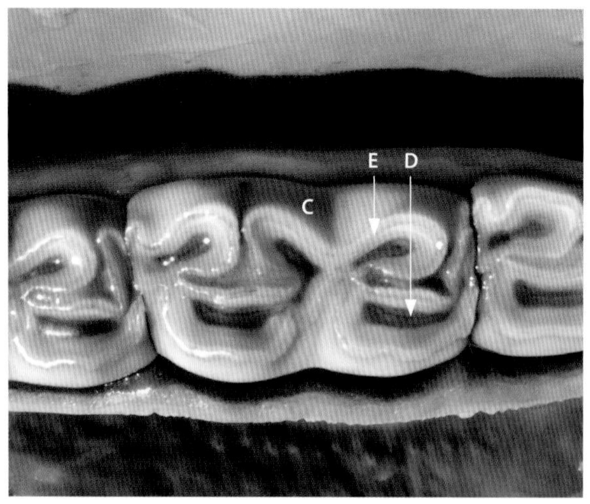

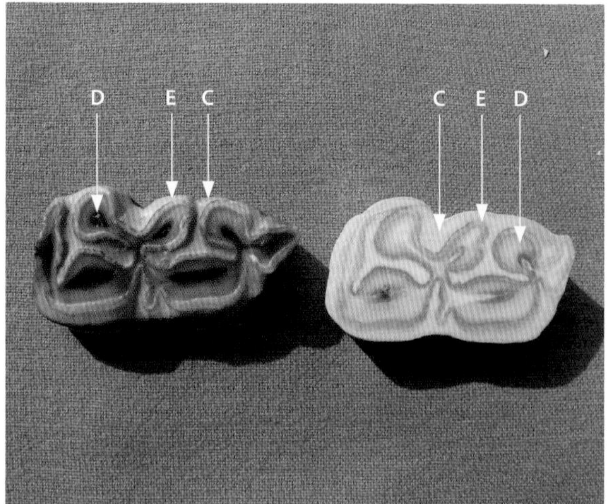

Top left:
View from above of the tables of the lower molars. The outer cream-colored layer is the cementum (C). The shiny white is the sharply twisting enamel line (E). The dentine is situated within this enamel line (D).

Above right:
A comparison between the table of a lower molar and a cross section of a lower molar sliced 1 cm below the table surface. (Left: the complete tooth. Right: the cross-section.) The various teeth components can now be clearly seen.

Illustration below:
A tooth is composed of cementum (C), enamel (E) and dentine (D).

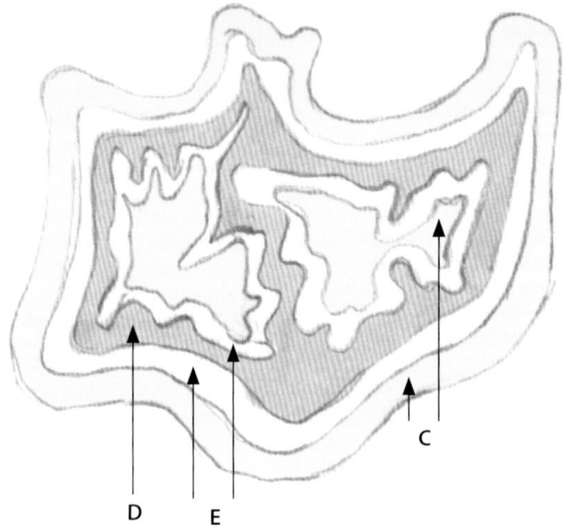

CHAPTER 4

Determining the Horse's Age

Throughout history, a horse's age has always been—and still is—a contributing factor in its market value. Whole books have been written about how to find out the age of a horse accurately by using the characteristics of its set of teeth. In the countries where obligatory identification of all horses is done by way of a microchip, the determining of age via the set of teeth has become less important. One can expect that eventually the endless debate about the ages of horses will be less frequent.

Determining the age of a young horse by its set of teeth is quite accurate. But from the age of 8 on, it can be considered more of an estimation of age and even then with a considerable margin: the older the horse, the less accurate the determination. The cutting of the milk incisors (teeth emerging through the gums in the mouth) and the replacement by the permanent incisors is quite fixed in time. Nevertheless, even here we see differences among breeds: the cutting of the milk incisors in the Shetland pony takes time while the replacement of the permanent incisors in a purebred Arabian is nearly six months earlier. The wearing down of the incisors with age however is distinctly individual. Variation is determined by breed type, fodder type, and any possible development of defects in the set of teeth that cause an abnormal chewing pattern and subsequently, abnormal wear and tear.

The following characteristics can be used to come to a conclusion about age; they are listed in order of reliability.

- Eruption of the incisors
- Changes on the surface of the table of the lower incisors
- Changes in form and angle of the incisors

Below left:
A full set of milk incisors in the lower jaw of a yearling.

Below right:
The lower incisors of a 4½-year-old horse. To determine age correctly, you can compare this set of teeth with that of the yearling pictured left. At first sight there are actually many similarities. Underneath at right (403) there is still a small milk incisor present; all the other teeth are permanent incisors.

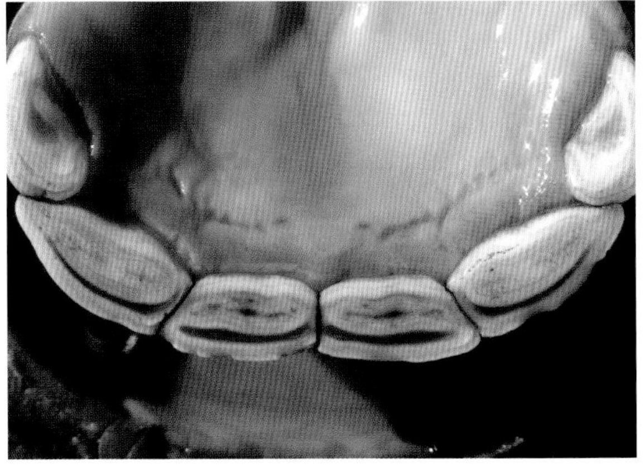

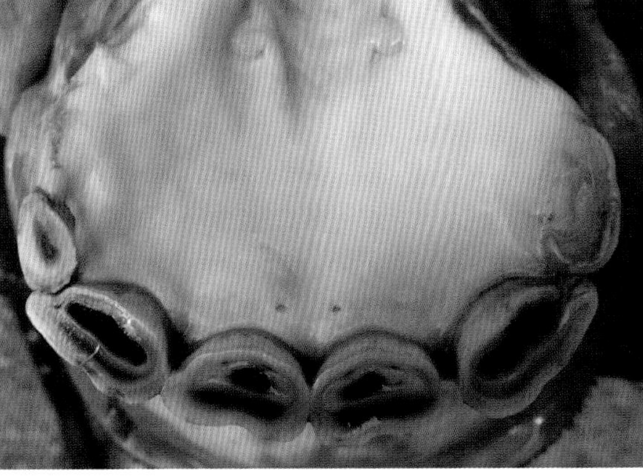

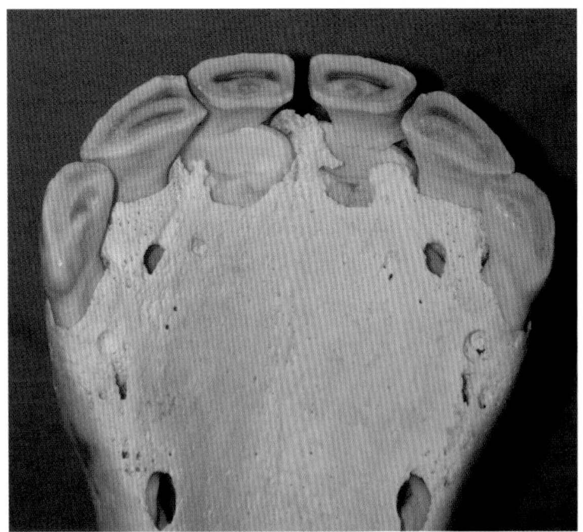

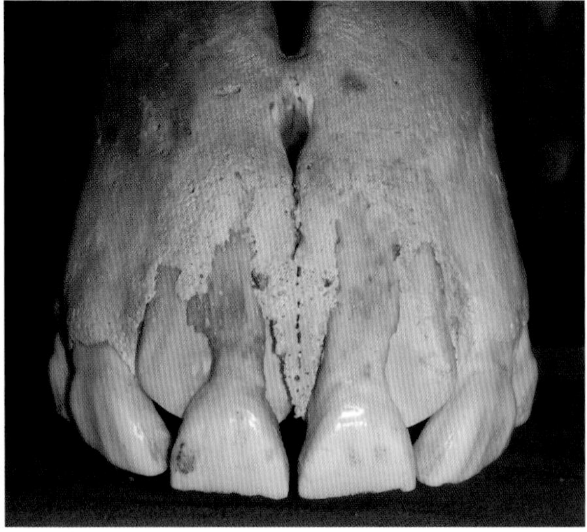

Left and right: Two pictures of the upper jaw of a skull of a horse of 2½ years old. The permanent incisors are in position to dislodge the roots of the milk teeth; the milk incisors will fall out in the mouth and the permanent teeth will grow through.

Eruption of the Incisors

The young foal cuts its central incisors (.01) during the first week of life, the lateral incisors (.02) at around 4 to 6 weeks, and the corner incisors (.03) at the age of 6 to 9 months. A good mnemonic is: 6 days, 6 weeks and 6 months. The replacement by permanent teeth follows similarly in the age order of 3 years old, 4 years old and 5 years old.

A yearling and an adult horse both have, nevertheless, a complete set of incisors so we must be able to see the difference between milk incisors and permanent incisors. The milk incisors are milky white and have a half-round visible crown. The permanent incisors have a more rectangular visible crown and have a more yellow tint due to the remains of the cementum. From the age of 5, the presence of canines in males clearly shows the difference between a young animal and an adult animal.

Changes on the Table of the Lower Incisors

a. The appearance of the dental star

The dental star appears on the lip side of the table in front of the mark at the age of 5 years old (.01), 6 years old (.02) and 7 to 8 years old (.03). Actually, this is the top of the root canal that gets filled with dentine as the wearing down of the incisor progresses. Dentine can absorb grass pigment and accounts for the yellowish-brown coloring of the dental star. When the dental star first appears it is line-shaped and parallel with the front of the incisor. In older horses, the dental star moves more to the center of the table and it also becomes rounder. However, if an individual horse, when young, had a root canal that came up nearly to the table, then the dental star would appear one or two years earlier than would

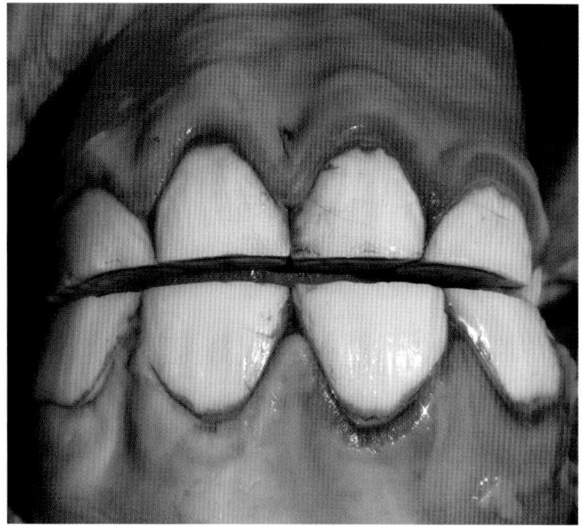

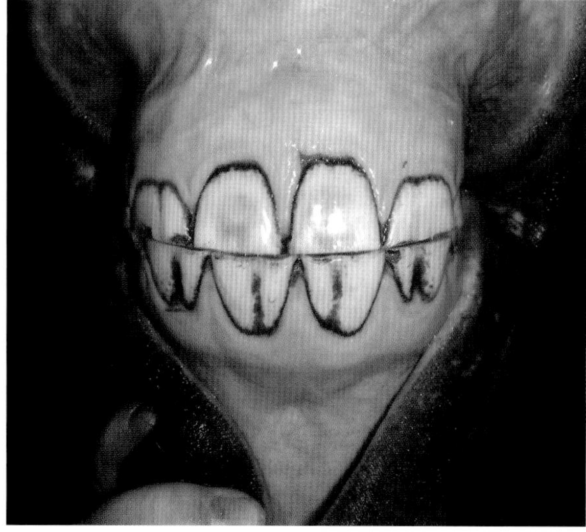

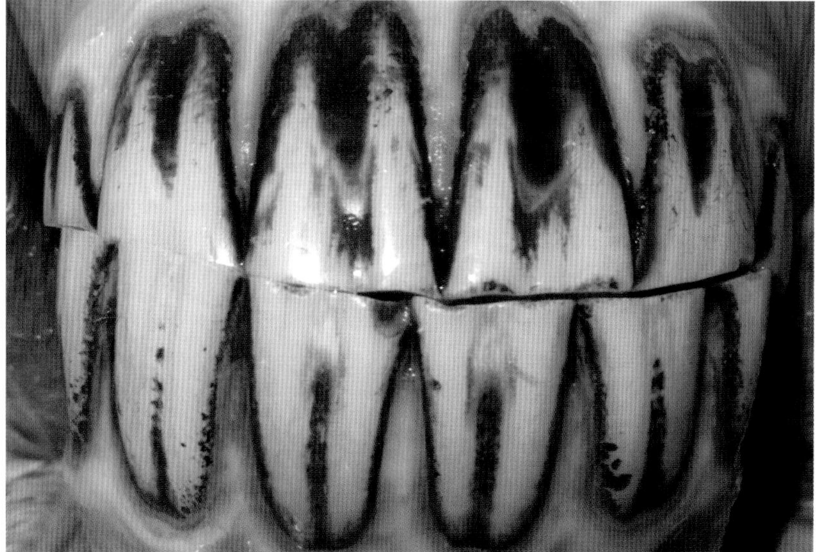

Top left:
Front view of the incisors of a yearling. The milk incisors have a half-round visible crown and are milk white and have no clear groove in their visible crown.

Top right:
Front view of the incisors of an adult horse of 6 years old. The permanent incisors have a more rectangular visible crown, are more yellowish-brown in color and have a groove in the visible crown.

Below:
In the older horse, the characteristics of the permanent incisors are even clearer: a more rectangular visible crown, yellow-brown in color, and a groove in the visible crown.

be normal. In horses older than 20, this is mostly the only characteristic left on the table.

In the center of the tinted dental star a white fleck appears. This occurs between 7 to 8 years (.01), 9 to 11 years (.02) and 11 to 13 years (.03).

b. The filling in of the base of the mark.

When the permanent incisor teeth erupt these have a depression (the mark). The mark gradually diminishes as the incisors are worn down by grinding; the mark completely disappears and it is then known as a "filled mark." A horse that has lower incisors where the mark has disappeared is known as "long in the tooth." It used to be thought that such horses were 8 or 9 years old. We now know that the age spread of "long in the tooth" is indeed much bigger, that is, 9 to 15 years.

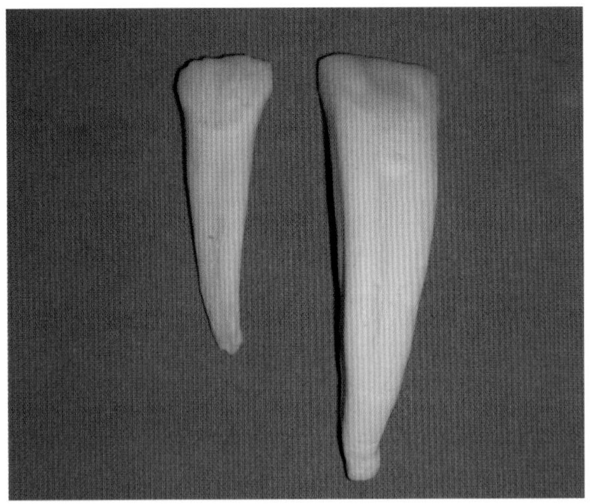

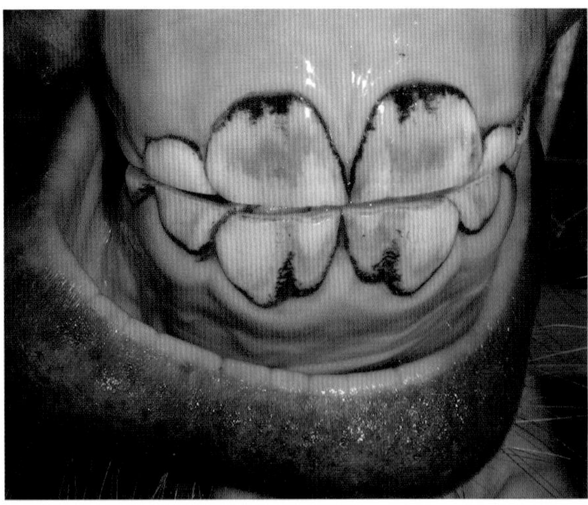

Above left:
The comparison in the size and shape of a milk incisor and that of a permanent incisor. The permanent incisor of a young horse can be up to 8 cm long. The milk incisor is smaller and has a more clearly marked, cup-shaped visible crown.

Top right:
The incisors of a 3-year-old horse. The central incisors have already been replaced. When milk incisors and permanent incisors are next to each other, it isn't difficult to see the difference: the permanent incisors are much bigger.

Illustration below:
In this diagram, the changes to the table are shown in the central lower incisors as the horse gets older (301 and 401). At 4 years old, the profile of the incisor is oval and there is still an obvious mark present. At 6 years old, only the remains of the base of the mark can be seen and the dental star appears on the lip side. As the horse gets older, the base of the mark disappears, the dental star comes more towards the middle and the profile of the table becomes rectangular.

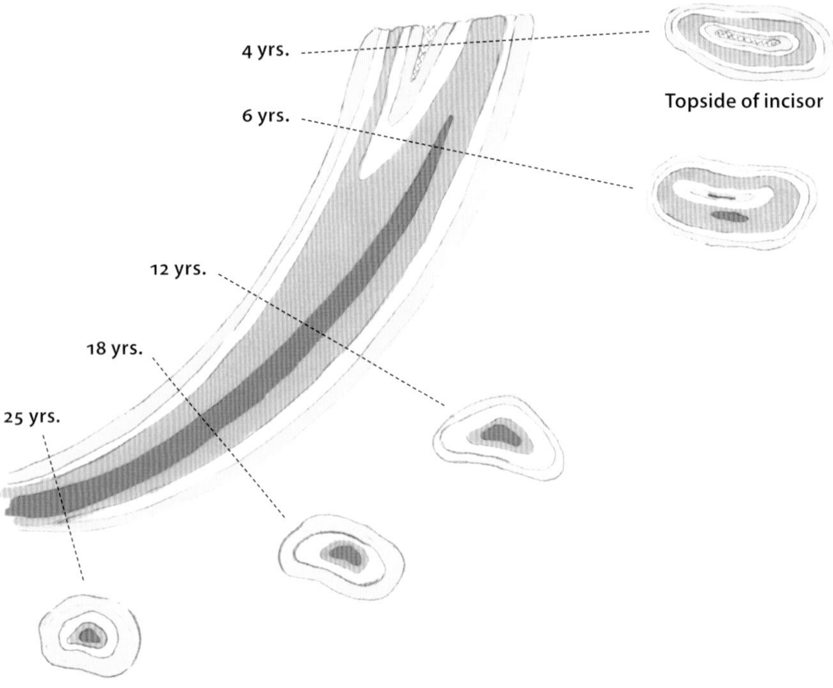

c. The disappearing of the remains of the mark base.

The shape of the table fairly well matches the shape of the mark base. In young horses this is oval; in older horses the shape becomes more and more round and is smaller. At about 20 years old, the mark base has completely disappeared from the incisor.

Changes in Form and Angle of the Incisors

In the young horse, the surface of the table of the incisors is oval and they fit fairly straight on top of each other. In the older horse, the table

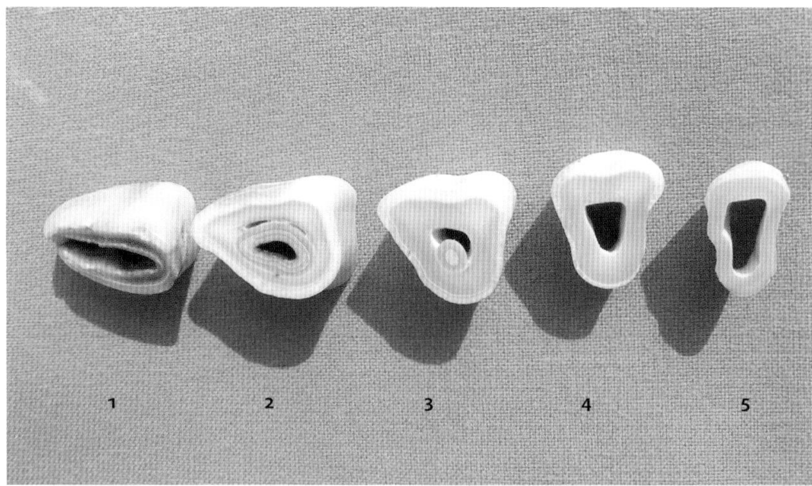

The cross sections of an incisor. At far left: the table. At far right: 1 cm above the root. In cross sections (1) and (2), the mark is visible. In cross section (3), the round remains of the base of the mark can still be seen. From cross section (2) on, the root canal can be seen. In the living horse, this root canal becomes filled with dentine during the wearing-down process. The dentine absorbs the pigment of forage and becomes visible as the brown dental star. Notice also the change of form on the outside of the incisor: as the horse ages, this form can also be observed on the table.

ultimately becomes triangular and the incisors fit on top of each other but at an oblique angle. These changes happen extremely gradually and they only give us a rough indication of age – for example, the indication of the age of a "very ancient" horse.

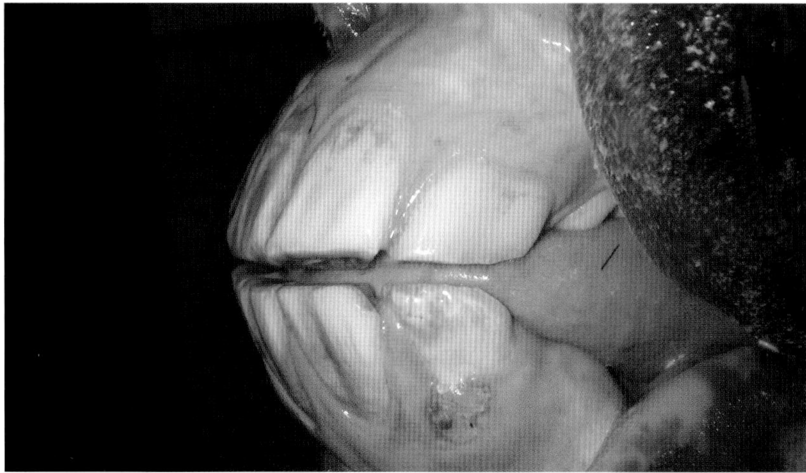

Left:
A side view of the incisors of a 5-year-old horse. The incisors are in a relatively upright position on top of each other.

Below left:
The incisors of a 12-year-old horse: the incisors meet at a more oblique angle.

Below right:
A side view of a horse "long in the tooth": in this case, 34 years old. The incisors clearly point forward.

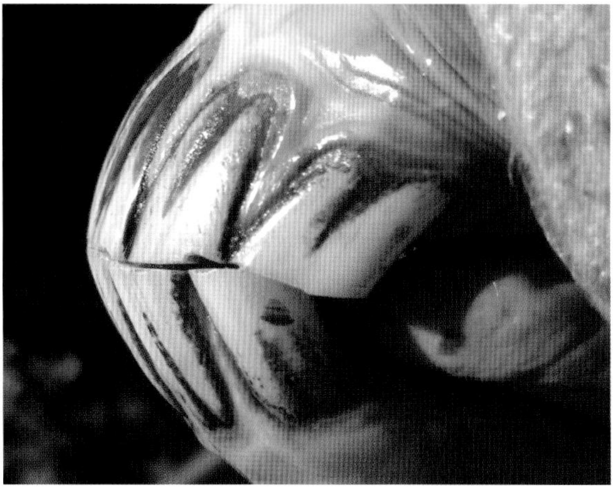

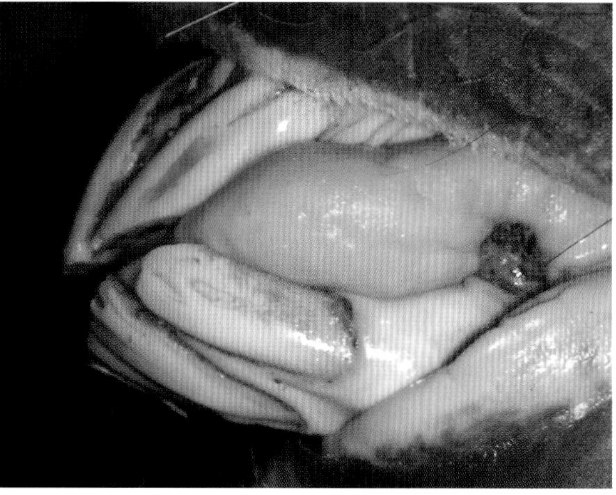

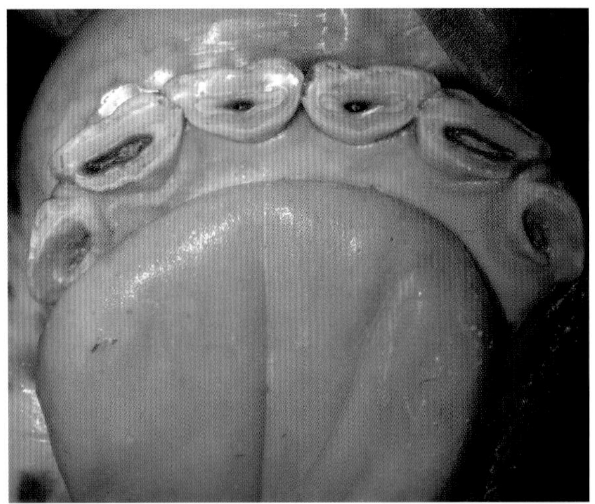

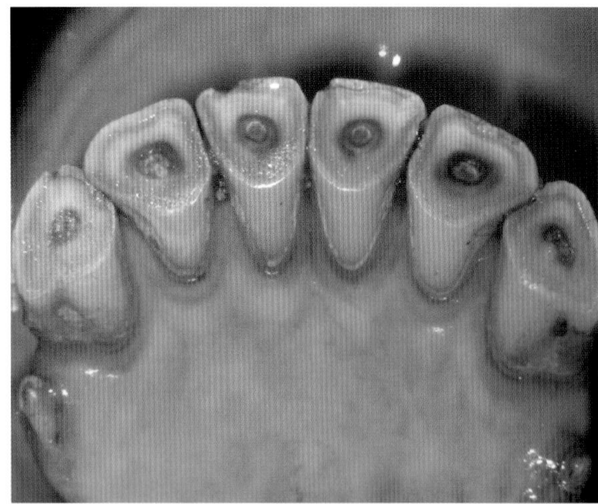

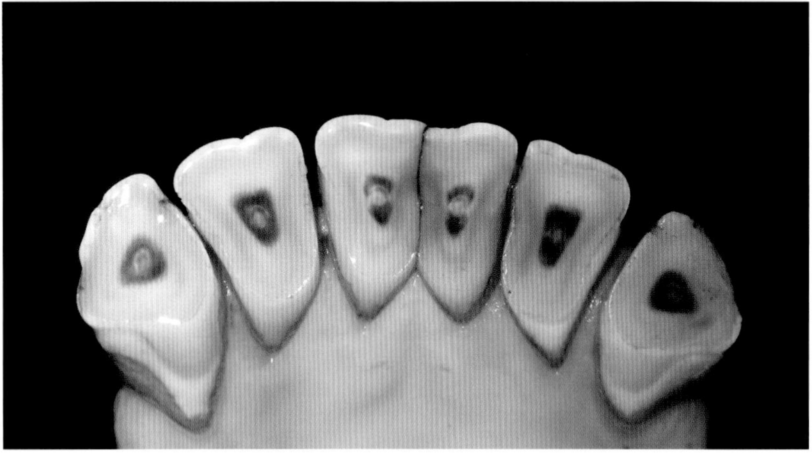

Top left:
The incisor tables of a 5-year-old horse are oval and form a line within the curve of the set of teeth.

Top right:
The incisor tables of an 18-year-old horse are more square-shaped.

Right:
The tables of the incisors of a 30-year-old horse are rather more rectangular.

Diagram of the eruption and replacement of the incisors

Determining age by the incisors	.01	.02	.03
Change to permanent incisors	3 yrs	4 yrs	5 yrs
Appearance of dental star	5 yrs	6 yrs	7-8 yrs
White zone in dental star	7-8 yrs	9-11 yrs	11-14 yrs
Filling in of the mark	6-7 yrs	7-11 yrs	9-15 yrs
Disappearance of mark base	~18 yrs	~19 yrs	~20 yrs

CHAPTER 5

The Chewing Cycle

The horse's set of teeth has evolved over time to grind an enormous amount of bulky, fibrous forage. Looking back historically, horses in the wild had to extract all their energy from the consumption of tough grass, roots and leaves. These horses had to graze for 16 hours a day to supply their energy needs. The modern horse with permanent access to fields still follows this same pattern. However, more and more horses no longer have the luxury of unlimited access to grass and instead are often kept stabled for nearly the whole day. These horses are then fed two or three times a day. As a great part of their rations consist of energy-rich concentrates, they do not need to chew very much in order to extract a great deal of their energy requirements. Many of our modern sport

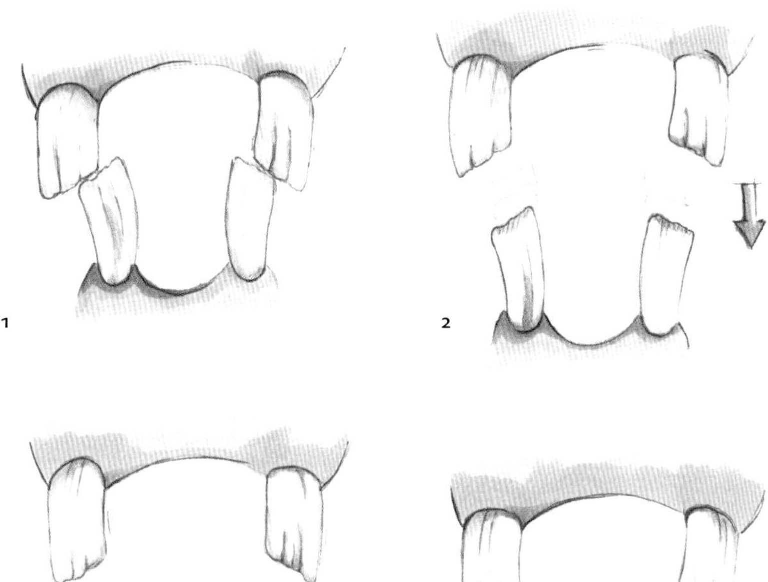

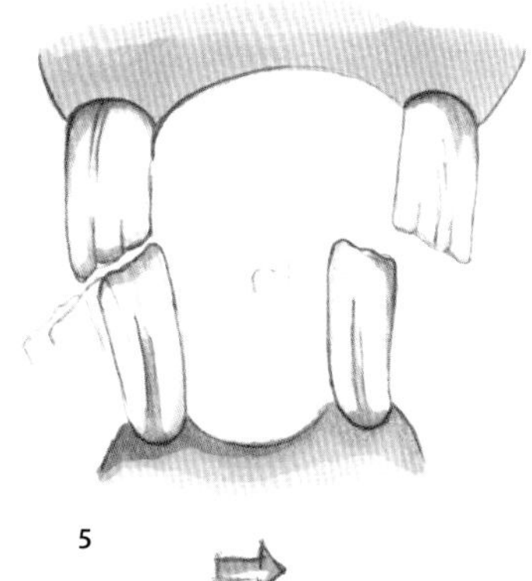

The chewing cycle. Initially, the teeth are at rest, positioned against each other (1). At the opening phase, the lower jaw is pulled away from the upper jaw (2). In the closing phase, the lower jaw returns with a sideways and upward motion (3 and 4). In the active grinding phase, the molars move with sideways pressure across each other whereby the forage in the mouth is ground (5).

Horses that are regularly put to grass usually have an even wearing down of their teeth as opposed to those horses that are fed mainly concentrates and hay. The chewing of grass produces a greater sideways movement of the lower jaw in opposition to the upper jaw.

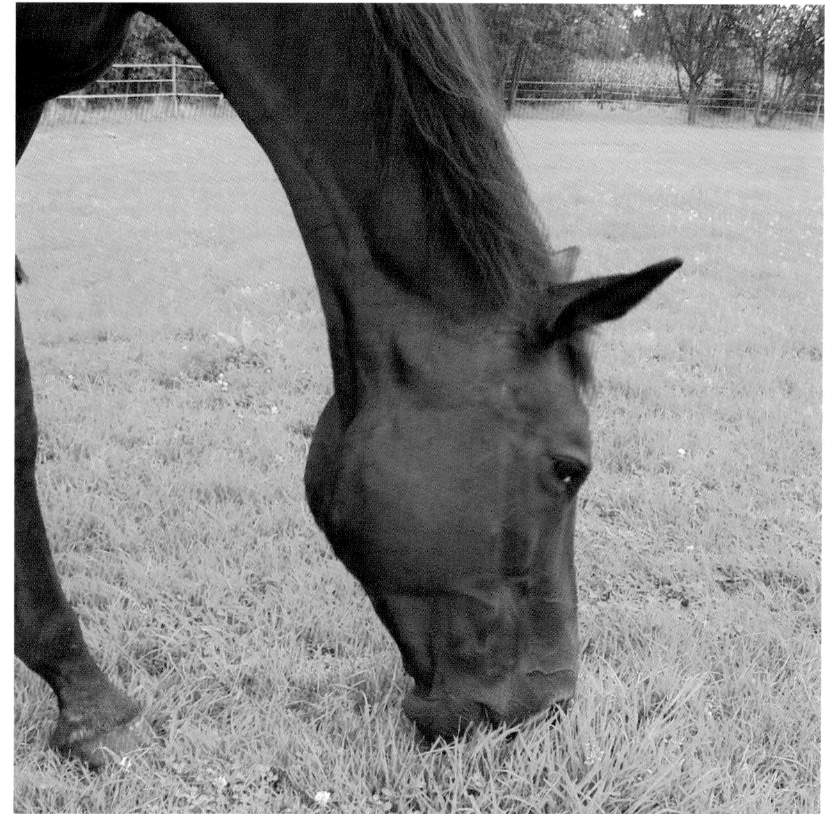

horses chew for only about three hours a day and this has enormous consequences for the degree of wear on the teeth.

Forage is tested and selected by the lips and drawn up between the incisors. The grass is pulled up with a short, nipping action and brought up into the mouth. As soon as a horse has a "mouthful" of forage, the grinding action of the molars commences. The tight cheeks and the up-and-down movement of the tongue against the palate ensure that the forage is deposited between the molars. The forage is worked towards the back of the mouth in a spiral-shaped ball. Once it has arrived at the pharynx it is then swallowed and the process of digestion begins.

The chewing cycle consists of three phases. In the opening phase, the lower jaw is pulled away from the upper jaw so that the molars are separated. In the closing phase, the lower jaw is moved sideways and upward. In the grinding phase, the lower jaw moves sideways back to the central position in order to grind the forage between the molars. Lastly, the jaw returns once again to the starting position.

There are 100 cycles per minute when grass is being eaten. If grass is replaced by hay, the number of cycles is reduced to 60 per minute. The degree to which the teeth move sideways is determined by the forage, that is, the amount of fiber and moisture present in it. Thus, when grass is eaten, there is a greater sideways chewing cycle than when hay is eaten. As grass has a far greater degree of moisture it is much easier to grind. Granular feed has the smallest sideways chewing cycle. It is thus clear that the eating of enough grass produces a better, and a more even wearing down of the whole grinding surface.

As has already been mentioned, the degree of wear on the teeth is determined by the strength and direction of the chewing cycle and by the size, shape and incline of the surface of the teeth, and by the composition of the rations. Painful conditions in the mouth or in the jaw muscles will lead to an abnormal chewing cycle. This would then cause an irregular wearing down of the teeth resulting in a vicious circle. Preventive dental care is aimed at precluding painful conditions and irregularities of the teeth by correction at an early stage. If you delay dental care until your horse can no longer eat then you are generally between five and 10 years too late in having the set of teeth restored to a functional whole.

CHAPTER 6

What Can I See When My Horse Has Dental Problems?

The answer to this is generally quite simple: nothing! Most horses suffer in silence. The fact that there is a lack of symptoms does not mean an absence of possible present dental disorders. It is when the actual disorder worsens that the horse sometimes shows signs that all is not well in its mouth. The only way to find out if there is something wrong is to look inside and feel around.

On the other hand, there are some signs displayed by the horse that do indicate there is probably a problem. The first group of symptoms appears when food is being eaten and chewed. A second group of symptoms is caused by problems noticed when a horse is ridden or driven.

If your horse displays one or more of the characteristics below and its teeth never have been thoroughly examined, it would be prudent to have a dental examination as soon as possible.

Considering that we really do not notice dental problems in most horses, a yearly dental inspection is most definitely advised.

Problems concerning food intake:

- A lot of concentrates (pellets or grains) falling out of the mouth
- Wads or balls of food being dropped ("quidding")
- Pulling faces at the start of, or during eating

Left:
Quidding (partially chewed lumps of hay being dropped from the mouth): this always indicates serious dental disorders.

Right:
The storing of food in the cheeks—squirreling—indicates a problem in one of the first molars.

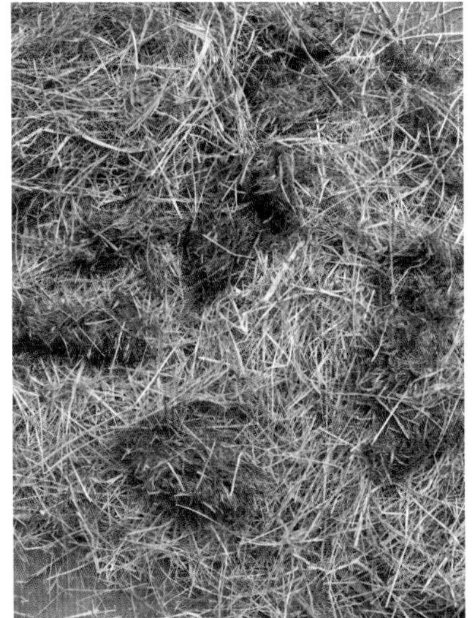

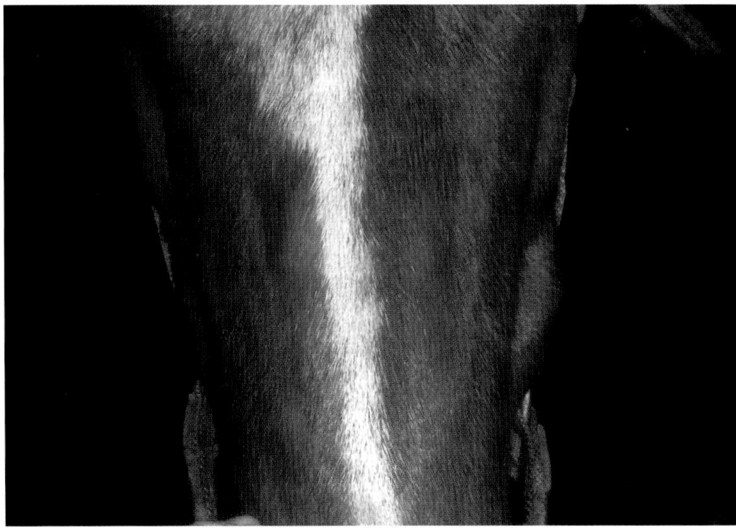

- Bad odor coming from the mouth or nose
- Raising the mouth in the air when eating
- Losing weight
- Many long wisps of hay in the manure
- Many undigested grains of feed in the manure
- Blockages in the esophagus and constipation colic
- Diarrhea
- Abundant saliva in the mouth
- Selective eating: eating grains but avoiding hay
- Squirreling: food in the mouth being stored in the cheeks

Problems concerning riding or carriage horses

- Difficulty in flexing to one side

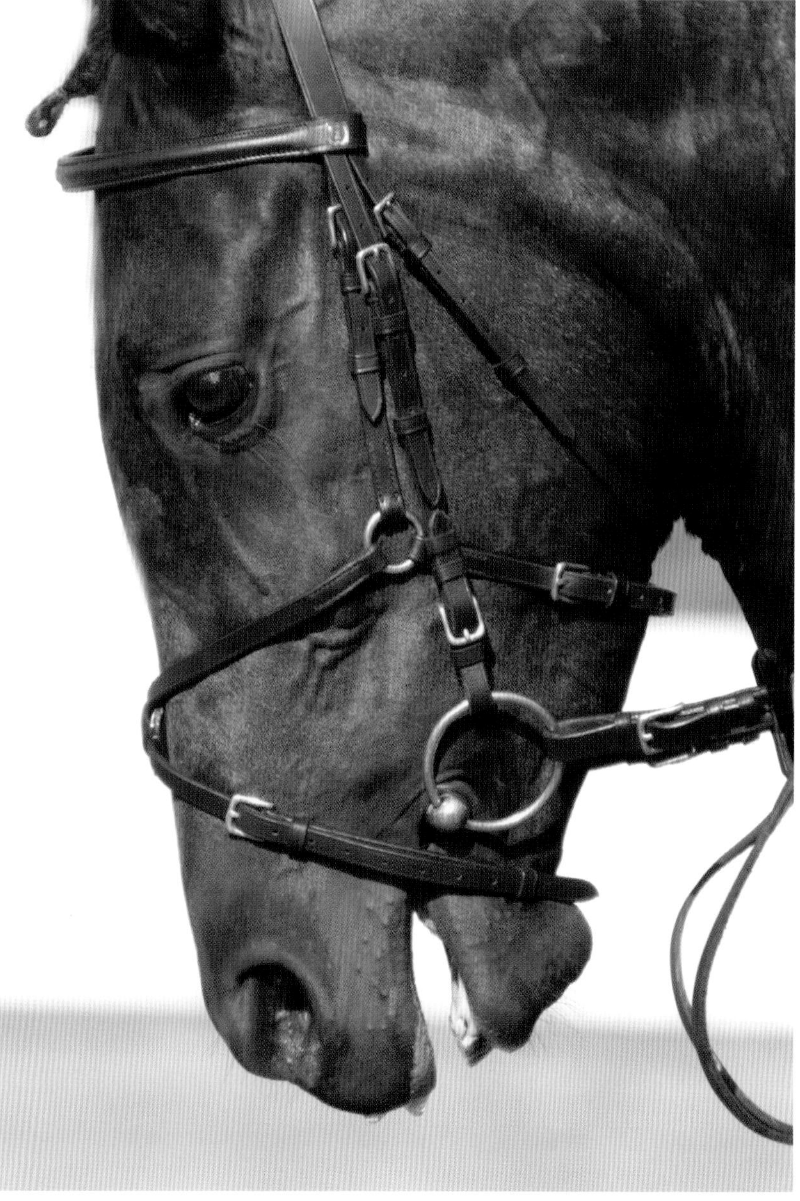

Going with an open mouth or other problems when riding on the bit can indicate a problem in the mouth. Note also the distressed look in the eye of this horse.

- Head throwing
- Continually playing with the bit
- Tongue hanging out of the mouth or being visible between the lips
- Blue tint of the tongue tip during work
- Rearing

Sudden changes when riding on the bit

- Head shy
- Can't be guided
- Tipping head to one side
- Pink tint to foam on the lips
- Unwilling to flex at the poll
- Sudden reluctance to maintain contact

Other problems

- A suppurating fistula on the outer surface of the head (see p. 77)
- Sinusitis: with or without pus running from the nose (see p. 76)
- A swelling on the outer surface of the head

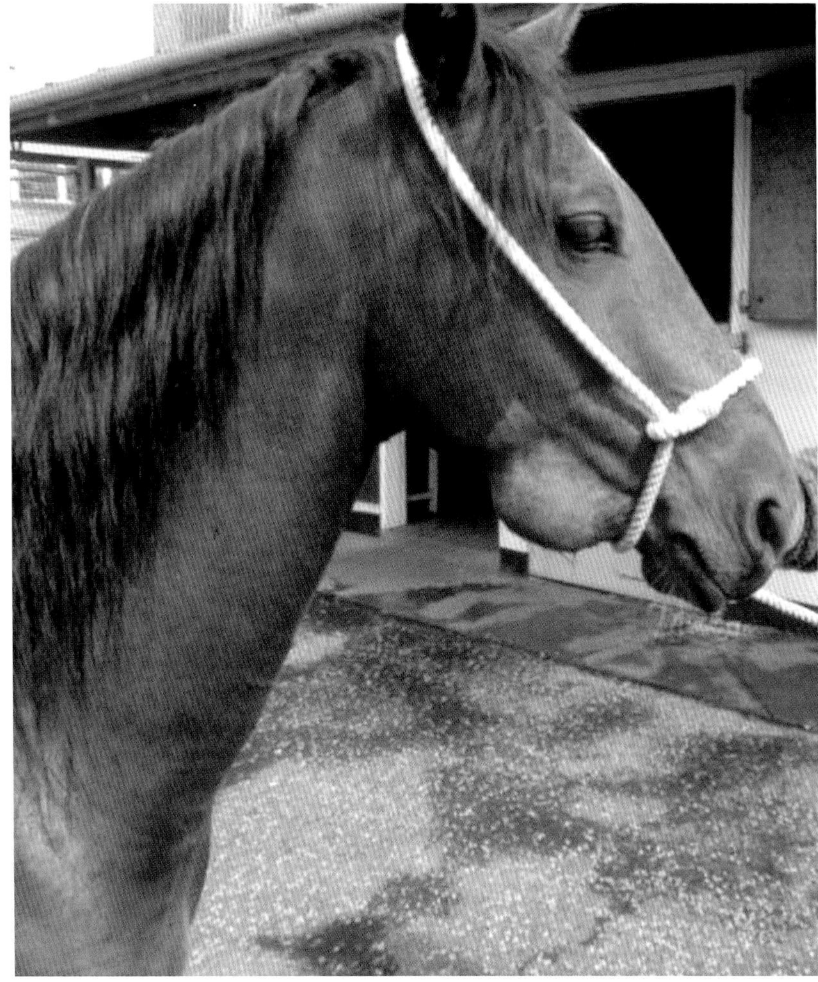

This horse has a very obvious swelling under its jaw which is caused by an infection in the root of the second molar. The infection has pushed through the jaw bone and an abscess has formed under the skin.

CHAPTER 7

Veterinarian, Equine Dentist or Dental Technician?

In most countries, "Equine Dentist" is not a title acknowledged by the various authorities and is definitely not what this name may lead one to believe: a qualified dentist who has become specialized in the care of horses' teeth. The term equine dentist is thus frequently and incorrectly used in the horse world. The words "dental technician for horses" would be a better description for both those people with a veterinary education and for those with another type of background. For this reason, in this book, I am using the term "dental technician."

Training

Veterinarians have studied disorders of the teeth and dental care for horses as a set part of the subject matter in their education. Formerly, this part of the education was rather limited and the chance to practice extremely scarce. Recently, however, there has been a clear attempt to improve the situation. The theoretical background was and is taught within the whole course of study: anatomy of the head, physiology of the digestion, the influence of the chewing apparatus on the digestion and so forth. Thus the veterinarian, at the level of the theoretical background, is in the ideal position to look after a horse's teeth. For the practical part, however, the saying "practice makes perfect" really matters: a veterinarian that only treats one horse a month will have difficulty getting enough practical experience skills.

Veterinary science is becoming more and more divided into specialities and today's equine veterinarians have enough horses among their clientele to gain the necessary experience that is required for the care of the teeth. The maintenance treatment of the horse's teeth can usually be quickly dealt with by such vets. Some veterinarians intensely dislike "doing teeth," which can lead to unpredictable results. Check with your own vet to see how he or she feels about dental care for your horse and whether or not the individual has enough experience. Some veterinarians have, after their training, gone on to further qualify in equine dental care by attending conferences, courses and apprenticeships at home and abroad of which these days there is an enormous variety.

The training of the dental technician that does not have a veterinarian's degree is, up to this day, very varied. Some have had a few weeks with a final examination. During this time a lot of theory is been covered and practical experience built up. The people who have completed the whole training can give a thorough examination of the horse's teeth and correctly carry out necessary treatment. However, others have merely done the basic course of a week and have not continued with further training. These people then advertise with flyers or via their Web sites that they have had such and such training at such and such school—and of course, they are not telling a lie. And, furthermore, other people produce seemingly impeccable qualifications that they've received from foreign institutes: institutes you can find no trace of however hard you search.

You should be most cautious with people who call themselves experienced "professionals." These people often just file away in the horse's mouth without the least bit of theoretical background in anatomy, physiology or possible pathological conditions of the mouth of the horse. Once I had a horse sent to me by one such person calling himself "experienced" with the urgent request that X-rays be made of the lower jaw of the horse because the bumps both on the left and the right on the underside of the lower jaw were apparently bone tumors. It concerned a four-year-old and I was able reassure the owner, without taking an X-ray, they were not tumors but normal mandibular bumps caused by the replacing of the second molar of the horse.

Guidelines

Many horse owners have never been in touch with a dental technician. This makes it difficult to make a well-founded choice. There are, however, a number of guidelines that can help: friendliness, smooth handling and being good with horses are good characteristics for a dental technician but, to this day, are not synonymous with professional competence.

A thorough dental examination as is described further in this book is a first requisite. What can't be diagnosed can't be treated. You should be able to expect an overview of actual disorders and what is proposed for treatment. Any dental technician can give you a final estimate of any necessary treatment after the examination.

Most disorders are possible to feel or see in your horse's mouth with the guidance of the dental technician. If feeling can be repeated after the treatment has been carried out, this ensures trust between the dental technician and you. A dental record of your horse with the defects and the treatment carried out allows you to monitor the development of your horse's set of teeth.

Editor's Note

In the United States, veterinarians perform dental work on horses, and laws pertaining to equine dental technicians vary from state to state: some states require a dental technician to have a veterinarian present for all tooth work; other states allow a technician to work with a veterinarian's approval; and there are states that allow a dental technician to administer basic dental care, floating teeth, for example. Specific information about the law is usually available online in a state's veterinary statutes. Two organizations: the International Association of Equine Dentistry (IAED) and the World Wide Association of Equine Dentistry (WWAED) qualify people through training and register technicians who have attended courses, fulfilled apprenticeship requirements, and passed examinations. Information about their members is available on their Web sites.

In the UK, the term Equine Dental Technician (EDT) is the correct term for a layperson who has shown skill and experience in dealing with certain equine dental procedures. The law in Britain on equine dentistry (covered in The Veterinary Surgeons Act 1966) clearly specifies which equine dental procedures lay people can perform and which can only be carried out by registered veterinary surgeons.

Currently in Britain a wide variety of lay people perform equine dental procedures. These vary from very inexperienced people, who have minimal training but nevertheless perform advanced dental procedures, sometimes damaging equine teeth. Other people (sometimes referred to as "tooth raspers") perform simple procedures such as rasping off small sharp dental overgrowths.

Only those people who have passed the British Equine Veterinary Association/British Equine Dental Association examinations are qualified to become members of the British Association of Equine Dental Technicians (BAEDT).

CHAPTER 8

Disorders of the Incisors

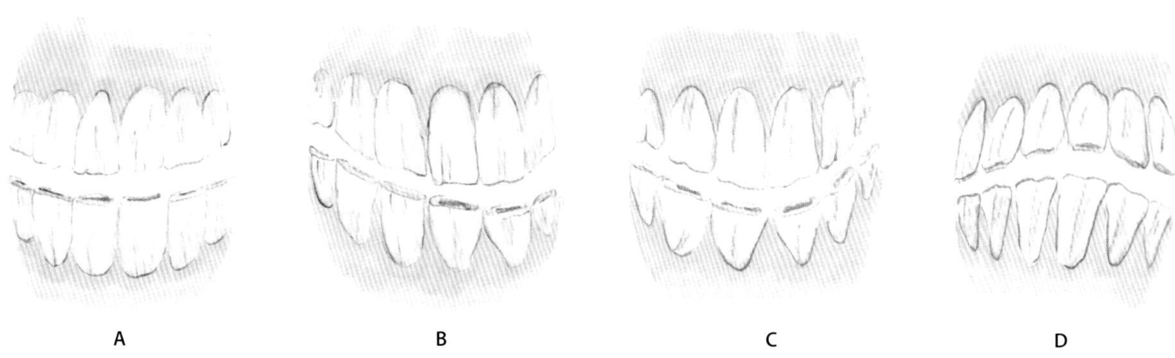

A. Normal incisors
B. Offset (diagonal bite) incisors: the upper incisors are longer on one side than the other: the reverse is the case with the lower incisors.
C. Ventral curvature: the central lower incisors are shorter and the lateral incisors longer so that a "smile" is formed, as it were.
D. Dorsal curvature: the central upper incisors are shorter and the lateral incisors are longer so that a "frown" is formed, as it were.

Step Incisors

When there is a "step" bite, there is a higher (taller) table on one or more of the incisors. This often occurs when an opposite incisor is missing or there is another disorder. A good sideways grinding movement is no longer possible because one table is higher than normal. Fortunately the taller table can be easily filed down.

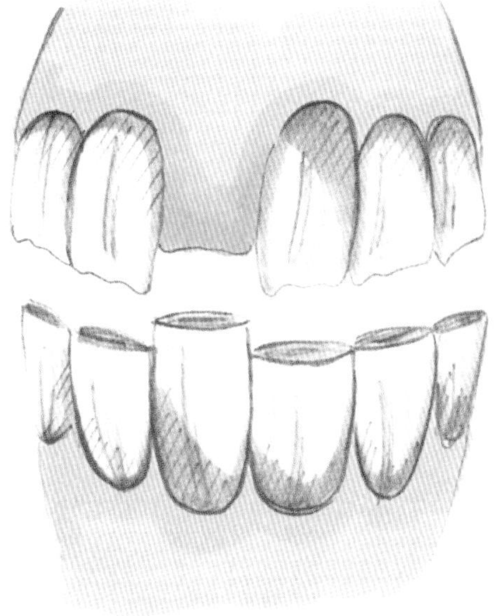

Step incisors. An incisor can be taller than the whole grinding surface due to insufficient or no wearing down of the table. This can impede or block the sideways movement of the jaw.

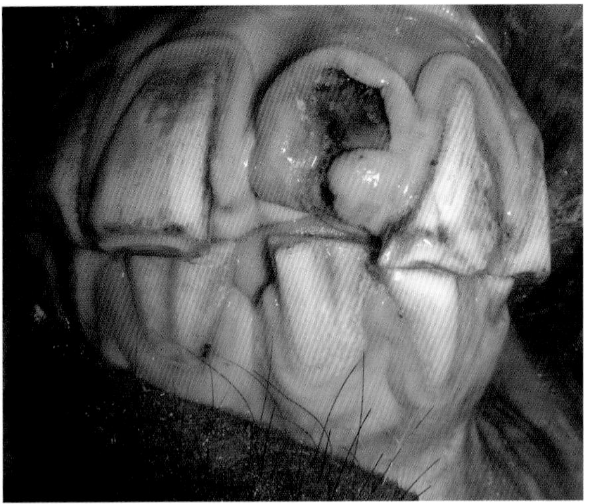

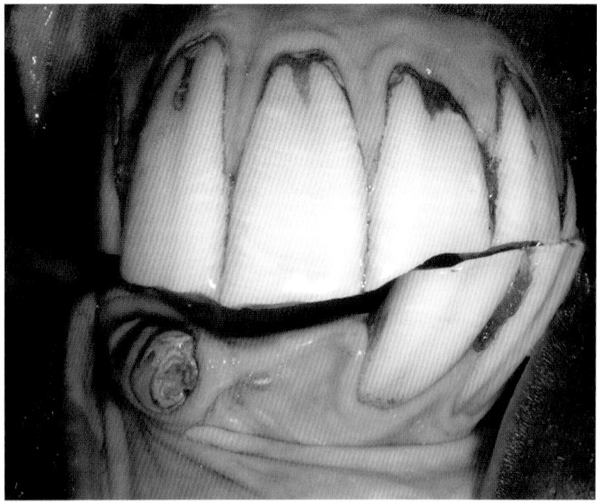

Top left:
Step incisor. This horse's incisor (201) was broken off by a kick from another horse some years ago. The opposite incisor (301) has, from lack of normal wearing down, grown up above the normal level into the space above.

Top right:
Step incisors. Due to three missing incisors (401 to 403: the broken-off root of 403 is still in situ) the opposite incisors have grown down into the space.

Ventral Curvature, Dorsal curvature and Offset bite

These are defects where all the incisors are involved. When we talk of ventral curvature, the upper incisors fit into the lower incisors in a downward bulge; the opposite occurs with a dorsal curvature—the lower incisors fit into the upper incisors in an upward bulge. In an offset or diagonal bite, the upper incisors are—on one side—longer than the lower incisors; the other side shows the reverse. This usually indicates a one-sided use of the jaw when chewing.

These defects evolve very gradually. Actually, the cause is unknown. It is possible that the different times of replacement of the opposite incisors may play a role but sometimes the defect can be purely attributed to an abnormal pattern of grinding. The correction is achieved by gradually reducing the higher side; sometimes this needs to be done in several sessions.

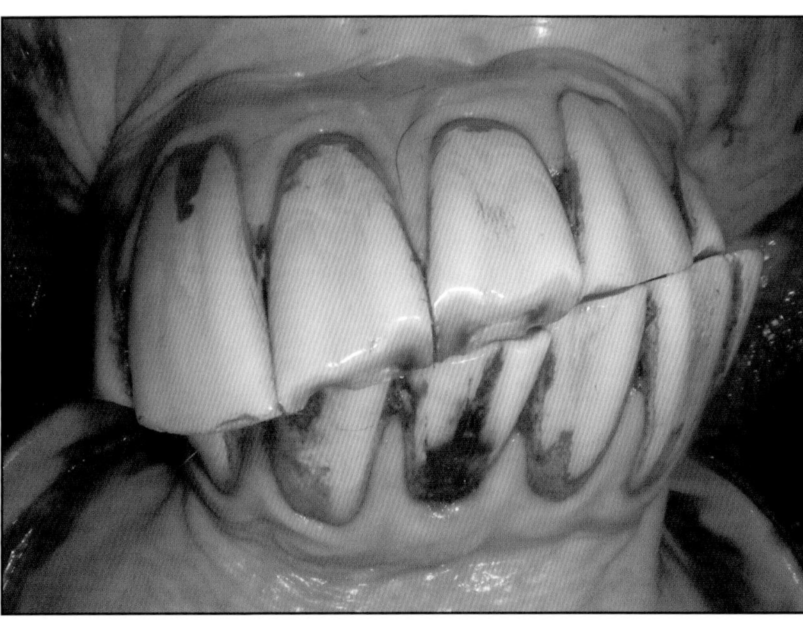

Offset incisors. The upper incisors are longer on one side: the reverse is the case with the lower incisors.

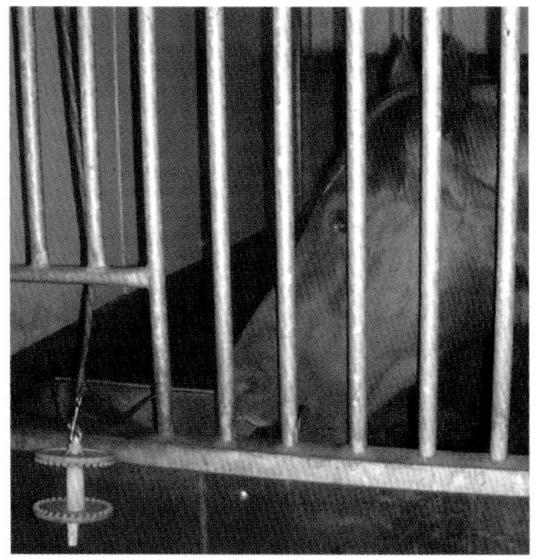

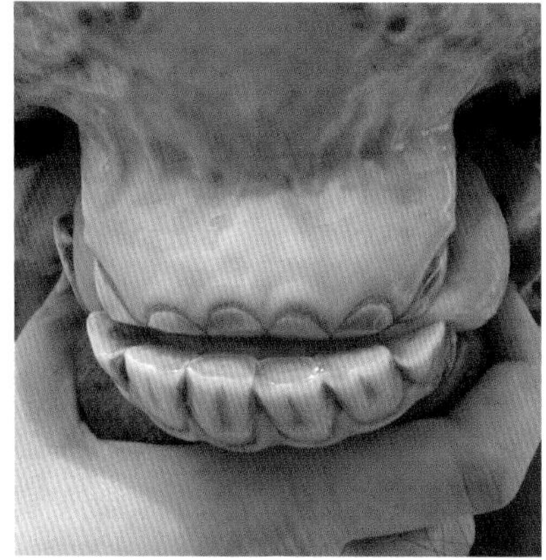

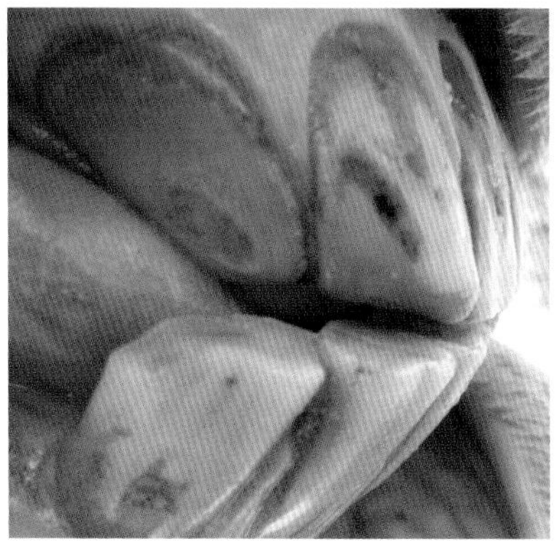

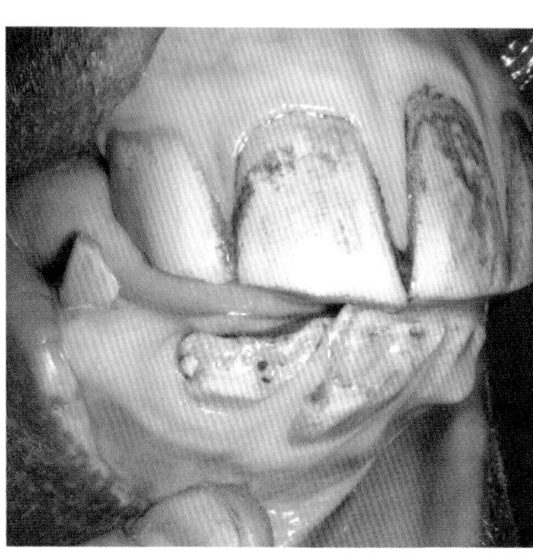

Top left:
When crib biting, the horse grasps a hard object with its teeth such as a manger and swallows air—a different vice called "windsucking." Often, in the long term, this leads to an abnormal wearing down of the incisors.

Top right:
This crib biter, and likewise windsucker, has nearly completely worn down the visible crowns of its upper incisors. Irregular wearing down like this is an indication that the horse is a crib biter and can be seen on examination at the time of purchase.

Below left:
The abnormal wear of this horse's upper incisors (102 and 103) is caused by the habit of dragging its teeth across the vertical bars of its stall.

Below right:
Abnormal wear of the lower incisors (402 and 403). This abnormal wear was caused by repeatedly rubbing them over a rough rail: tiny bits of the incisors continually broke off.

Crib Biting

In this stable vice, the horse grasps the feed bucket or manger, or a similar hard object such as the door, with its incisors. This often goes hand in hand with swallowing air at the same time. As the horse does this exactly the same way each time, there is often abnormal wearing down of the front of the table of the incisors. Deforming its teeth this way seldom causes problems for the horse. And it is easy determine in an examination at time of purchase.

Long Incisors

These days it is often recommended that incisors that are too long be cut back. When an extensive correction of the molars has taken place such as the trimming of a large rear hook or a "wave" bite, it is possible that the molars have been reduced by so much that the incisors have thus become relatively too long; this results in the molars having no contact when the horse is chewing. In such a case, it is best to shorten the incisors. However, a major correction of the teeth such as this is seldom performed.

Nevertheless, more and more routinely the table of the incisors is treated either by reducing or changing the angle of inclination. In the United States, a formula for the ideal set of horse teeth with the accompanying margins has been drawn up: every set of horse teeth is meant to meet with this standard. Even when there are no clinical problems present or to be expected, an endeavor is made to reduce the incisors to conform to this ideal definition.

I would very much like to add my comments to the above. There is also an ideal set of teeth described for humans as well, but who has such a set of teeth? The extent of the contact of the tables between the upper and lower teeth is mostly examined when the horse is under an anesthetic. The active impact that the massive chewing muscles have when coming together has then in no way been taken into consideration. No living creature—including humans—has the grinding surfaces of their molars in contact when at rest. What I think even more important is that at this time there is no scientifically proven basis for this manner of treatment. Any real advantage for the horse has not yet been proved despite the attractive theory built up for the reduction of the incisors that is cited.

Top:
This illustration depicts a "persistent" milk tooth. This is a milk tooth that has not fallen out in time and so it prevents the correct position of the permanent incisor from happening.

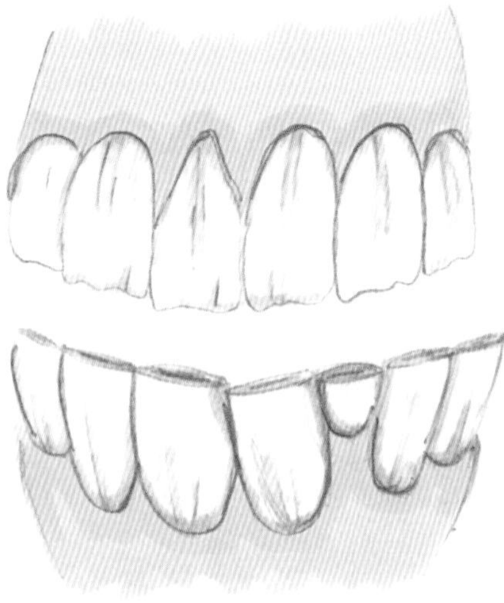

Below left:
The persistent milk tooth prevents the permanent tooth from filling its proper position among the other incisors. Removal of the persistent milk tooth will create space for the permanent incisor; this can then push forward and take its position in the row of teeth.

Below right:
This 8-year-old has a persistent milk tooth between two permanent incisors (402 and 403). It has caused the lateral incisor (403) to be positioned too far back and there was a vertical hook due to the absence of normal wear from the opposite incisor at the back of the table. This hook was radically corrected seeing that this disorder would definitely arise again in the future and that part of the table was not functional, anyway. Removal of persistent milk teeth at this age is no longer useful: the eruption of the permanent incisors has been completed.

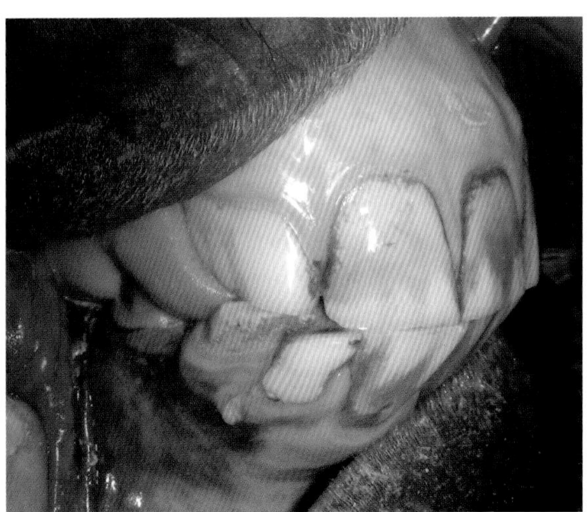

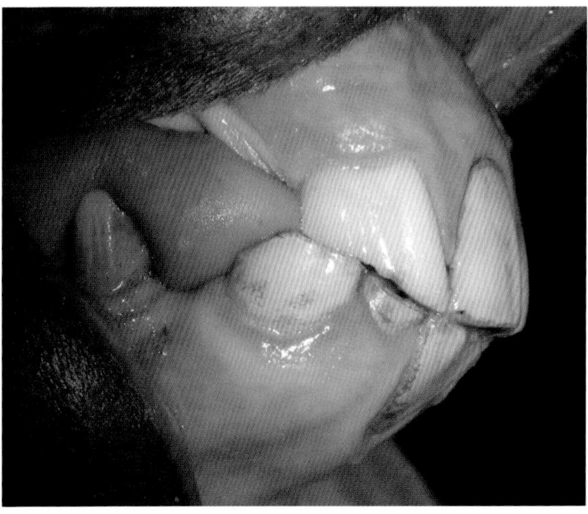

For the time being, then, my advice is to be cautious when there is a question of reducing "normal" incisors. Only when there are disorders as described above is correction scientifically justified.

"Persistent" Milk Incisors

When the milk teeth are replaced, milk roots are squeezed and wasted away by the pressure of the erupting permanent incisor. The remains of the crown fall out of the mouth when the permanent incisor erupts. Sometimes the permanent incisor erupts through at the tongue side of the milk incisor, in which case the root of the milk incisor is not destroyed and the milk tooth remains within the incisor arc. This results in there being no room for the permanent incisor in its proper position in the incisor arc. In the long term, this can lead to less wearing down on the table of this tooth and the normal sideways grinding mechanism could be reduced. To prevent this situation, the milk incisor concerned can be extracted so that the permanent tooth can take up its correct position in the space created.

Tooth Fractures

Sometimes an incisor is broken by a kick from another horse or other such trauma; this is less likely with the molars. In brachydont teeth—such as found in humans—the accidental opening of the root canal always leads to the loss of the tooth. This is not always the case with horses. Some horses even overcome the infection of the root canal and the root canal is sealed off from the outside by dentine. Root canal treatment can be carried out in the case of an incisor with an opened root canal. The root canal is cleaned and filled with synthetic dental material.

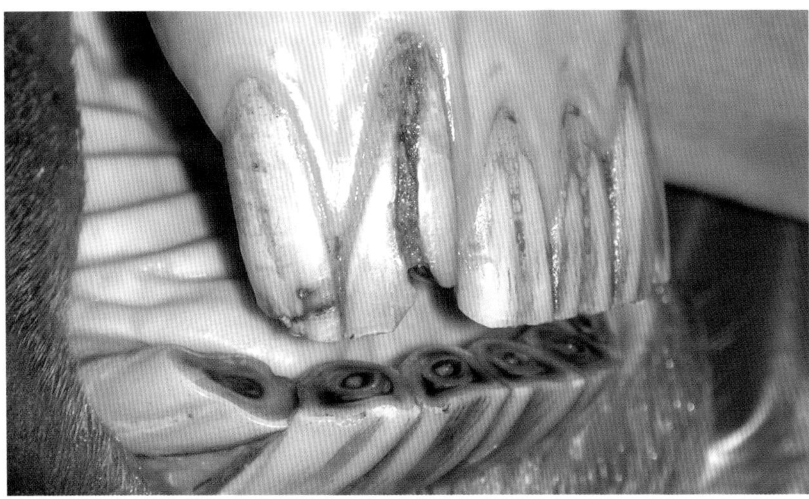

This incisor (102) was broken the whole way up to the root; it was confirmed by X-ray. The crack was packed with food. The only possible treatment was to remove the whole incisor.

Tooth Socket Fractures

It is mainly young horses that have the tendency to take things into their mouths such as a length of rope or fencing. Sometimes, while making an unexpected movement, things get caught in their teeth and in the process of pulling free, the teeth and part of the socket are pulled out. In the acute stage, there can be a lot of bleeding. The horse can usually still eat so the wound becomes covered and contaminated with food. You should always endeavour to save the teeth. After a thorough cleaning, the teeth together with their sockets are put back in place and fixed to the other teeth by metal surgical thread. After four to six weeks the metal brace is removed and the problem is solved.

Top:
This illustration depicts a tooth socket fracture. Here, the socket has broken away from the jaw together with several incisors. This sort of injury is seen mostly in young horses that get hold of a rope, for example, and then there is a sudden unexpected movement that causes the fracture.

Below left:
A tooth socket fracture. This 2-year-old stallion got his upper milk incisors (102, 101 and 201) caught in something and the socket around these incisors was fractured. At the time of presentation the fracture was clearly contaminated with food.

Below right:
After administering tranquilizers and a local anesthetic for the whole upper arc of incisors, the wound was cleaned and then thoroughly rinsed and disinfected.

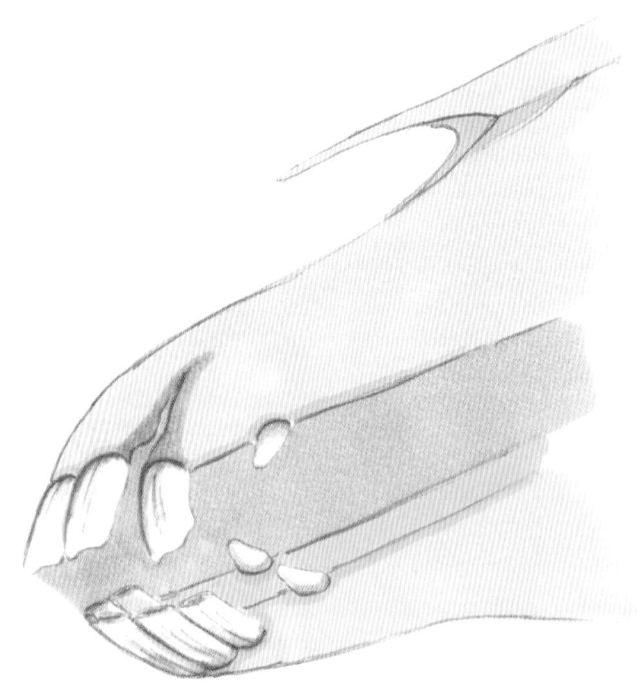

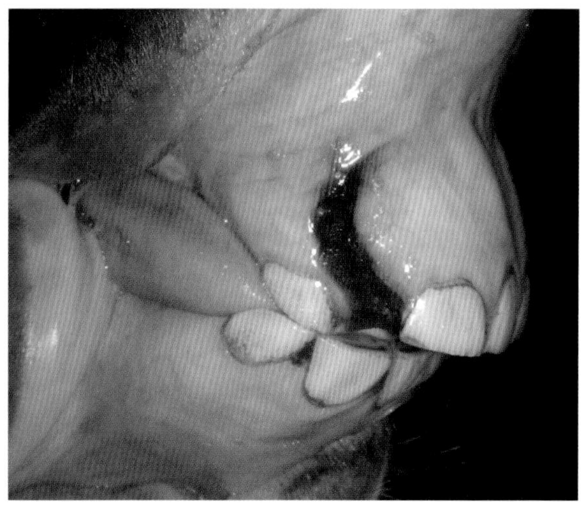

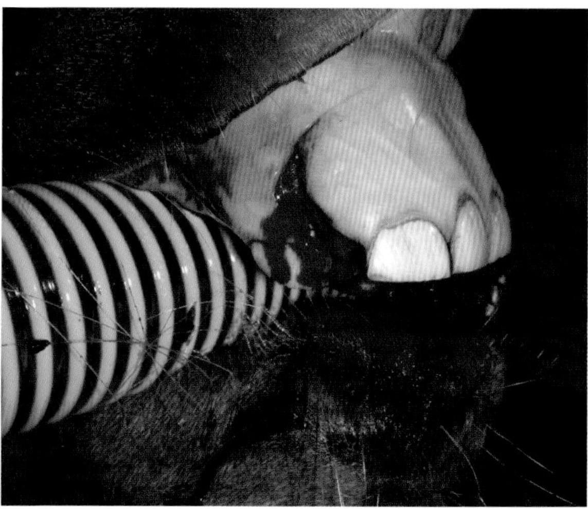

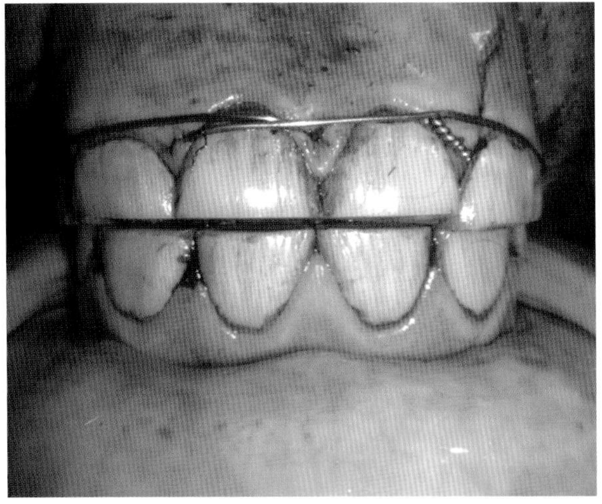

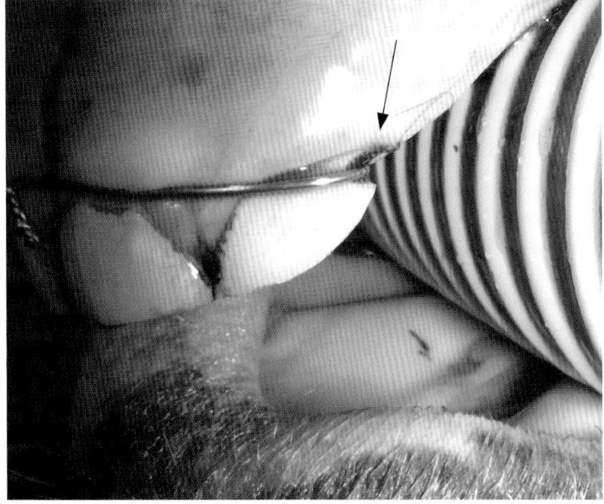

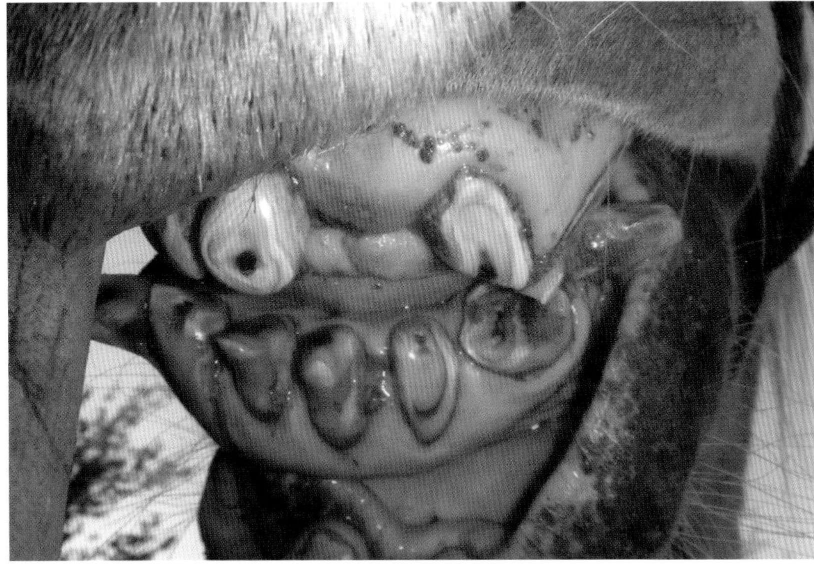

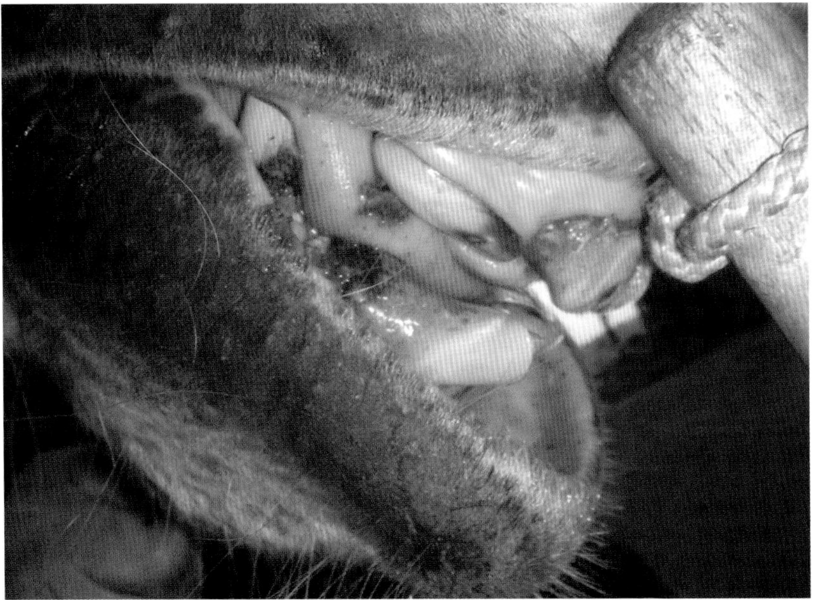

Top left:
Subsequently, the incisors, together with the bone, were set in place with metal surgical thread and fixed to the corner incisors. The tables of the incisors concerned were lightly cut back to reduce the pressure of chewing on the incisors and bone.

Top right:
In order to prevent the metal thread from slipping, a small groove was filed into the corner incisor. After eight weeks, the fracture was healed and the metal thread could be removed.

Middle and Below:
These are the incisors of a horse that, according to its owner, "had something happen to its head once." Notwithstanding that the incisors are all over the place and there are several abnormal tables, this horse showed no symptoms of dental disorder and was in good general condition. The teeth show no abnormalities in their wear, which is quite remarkable considering the state of the incisors.

CHAPTER 9

Disorders of the Canines

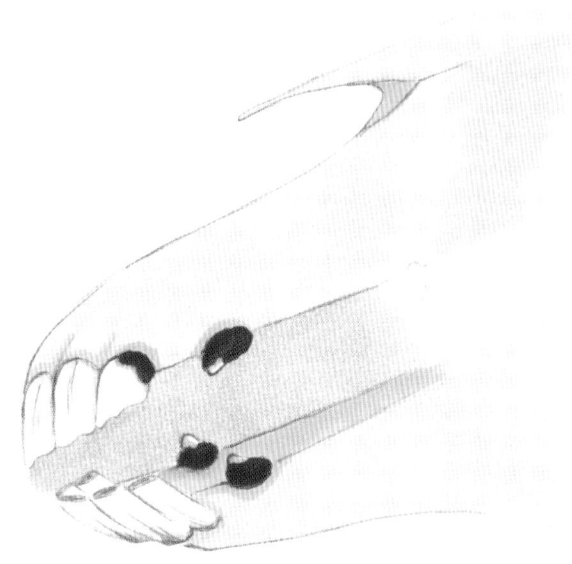

Plaque deposits in the older horse are seen mainly round the canines and, somewhat later, on the corner incisors.

Plaque Deposits

Plaque consists of an organic structure where minerals are deposited and it is a yellow-brown color. Plaque is often seen in older horses on the lower canines and on the lip side of the corner incisors. The canines are not used for taking-up or grinding forage, therefore they are not continually being "polished" by rough forage as occurs with the other

Below left:
Only the point of the canine is still visible under the thick layer of plaque. The plaque deposit is usually quite smooth on the outside.

Below right:
Irritation round the canine gum is clearly visible after removal of the plaque deposit.

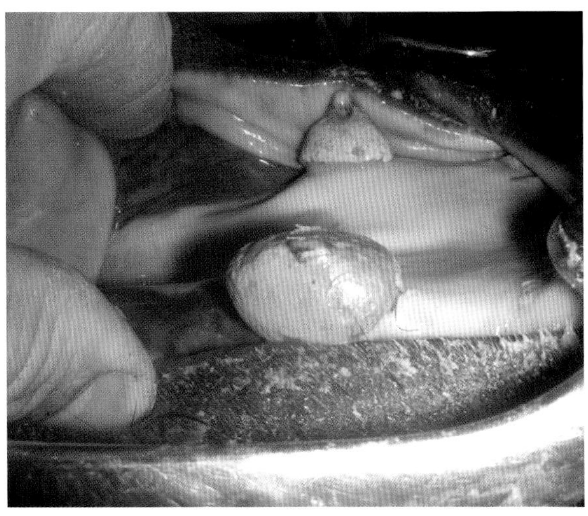

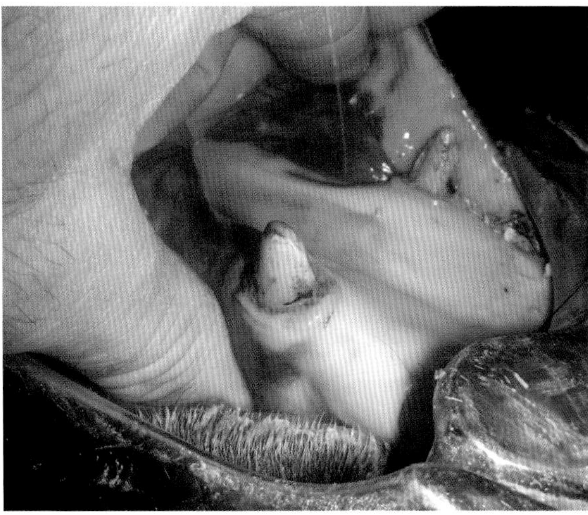

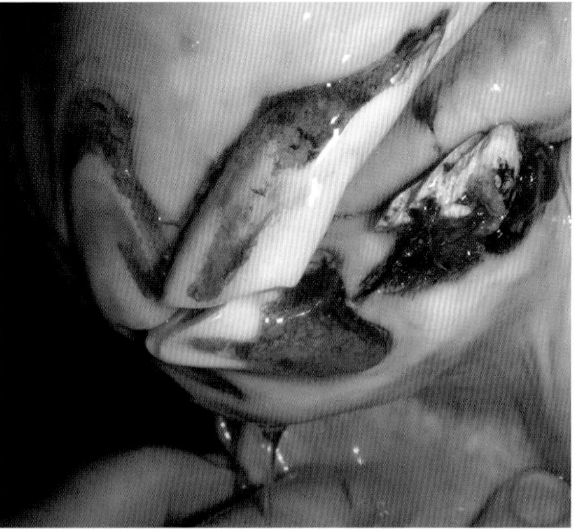

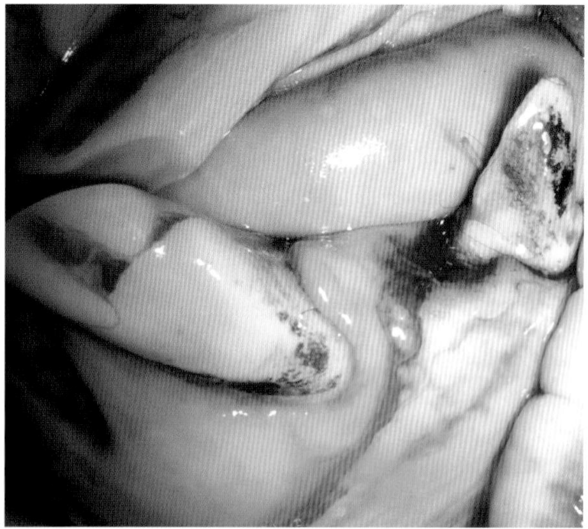

Top left and right : Sometimes the outside of the plaque deposit round the canine is peculiar in form. When this plaque was removed there was even some spontaneous bleeding.

Below left and right: Sometimes the canine is no longer visible under its strangely shaped deposits. In this older horse there were also light plaque deposits on the incisors. The difference between the left and right canine is now enormous. Notice the dark red swelling of the gum at the base of the canine. In the center of the picture on the right, you can see the plaque deposit that was removed.

teeth. Moreover, the submandibular salivary gland discharges into the mouth on the inner side of the lower canines. This is why the building blocks for plaque deposits are fully present at this spot. The underlying gum is often rather swollen and bleeds easily. Plaque is seldom the cause of any real clinical problems, and can be removed at the time of the dental checkup.

Sharp Canines

Canines can sometimes be very pointed. Nevertheless, I rarely see irritation or injuries on the side or underneath the tongue caused by pointed canines. Some dental technicians trim the canines to prevent their arms from being cut or injured while they examine the horse's mouth: I have never had this happen to me. If one of your horse's canines has to be reduced, it is best done so that it is level with the height of the corner

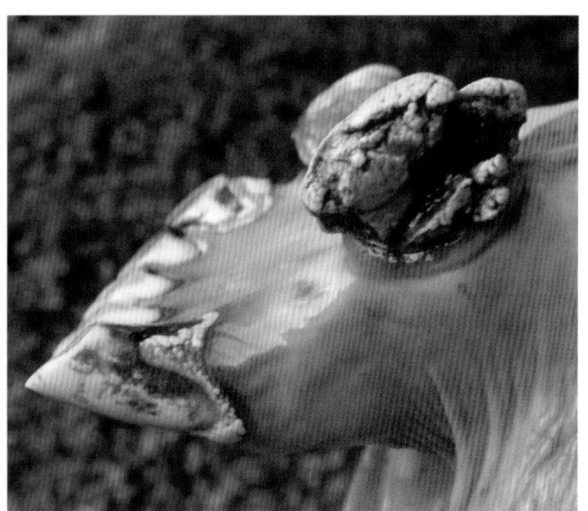

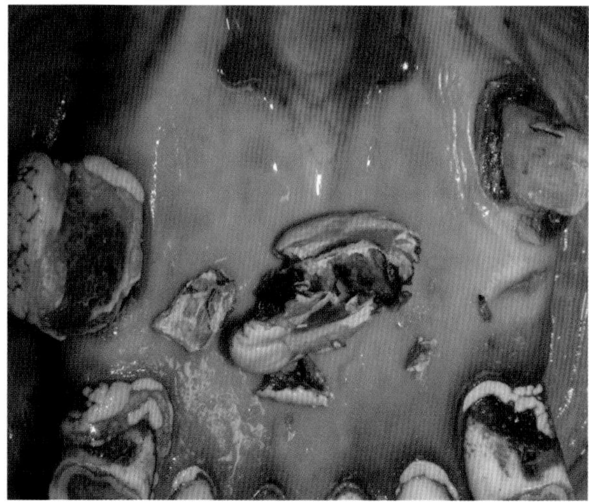

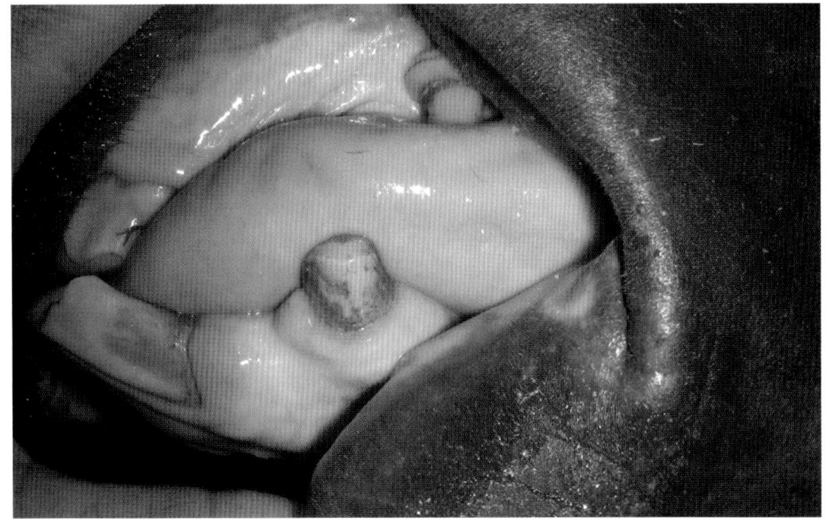

Sometimes canines that are too sharp are reduced and rounded down to prevent injury. As a guideline for reducing, the back edge of the table of the corner incisor is taken as the level.

incisor. Never let your horse's canines be filed down to the level of the gums: there is a risk that the root canal will be filed open with the possible chance that, eventually, the canine will die as a result. An additional risk is that the horse will hang its tongue out in the spot where the space has been created.

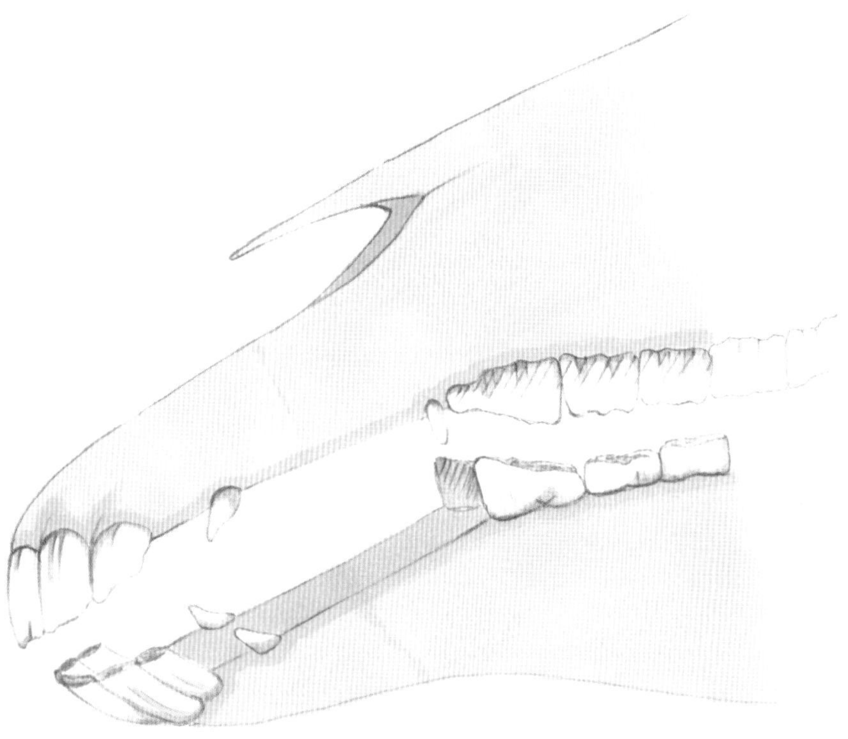

Canines that are too sharp may sometimes cause injury to the tongue.

CHAPTER 10

Disorders of the Bars

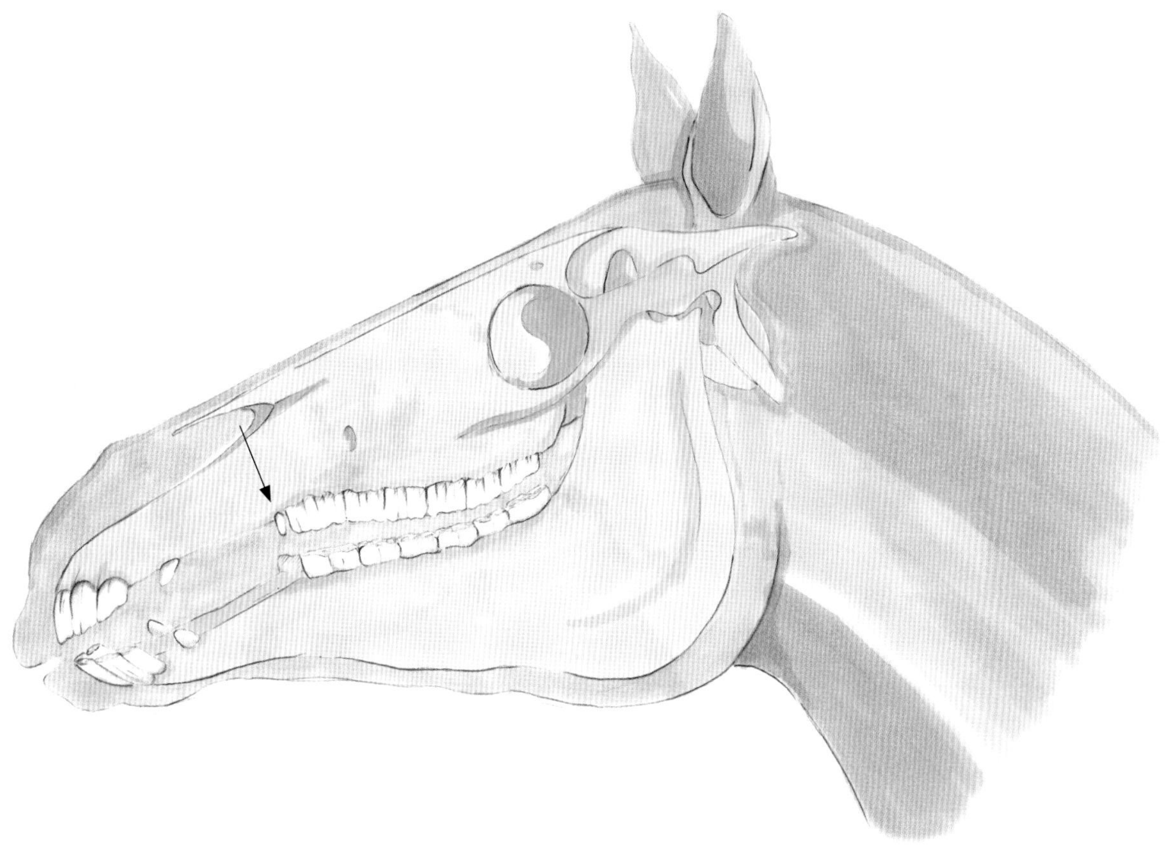

Wolf teeth are situated just in front of the first molar

The Wolf Teeth

Wolf teeth (.05) are present in about 25 percent of horses. They are mostly seen in the upper jaw just in front of the first molar; they are seldom seen in the lower jaw. Unlike the other teeth in the horse's mouth, these are brachydont teeth. As soon as they appear, they do not continue to grow and they have a short crown in relation to the root. They are usually only about 1 to 2 cm in length and they only show a couple of millimeters above the gums.

Actually these teeth don't really belong in the list of dental disorders seeing that they cause no problems in horses that are not ridden. It is only when a bit is put in the mouth that there is a possibility of problems being caused by the wolf teeth. The stability of these small teeth in their sockets can be put under pressure by the bit and the teeth can sometimes even break off. When the wolf teeth are absent, the pressure from the bit rests

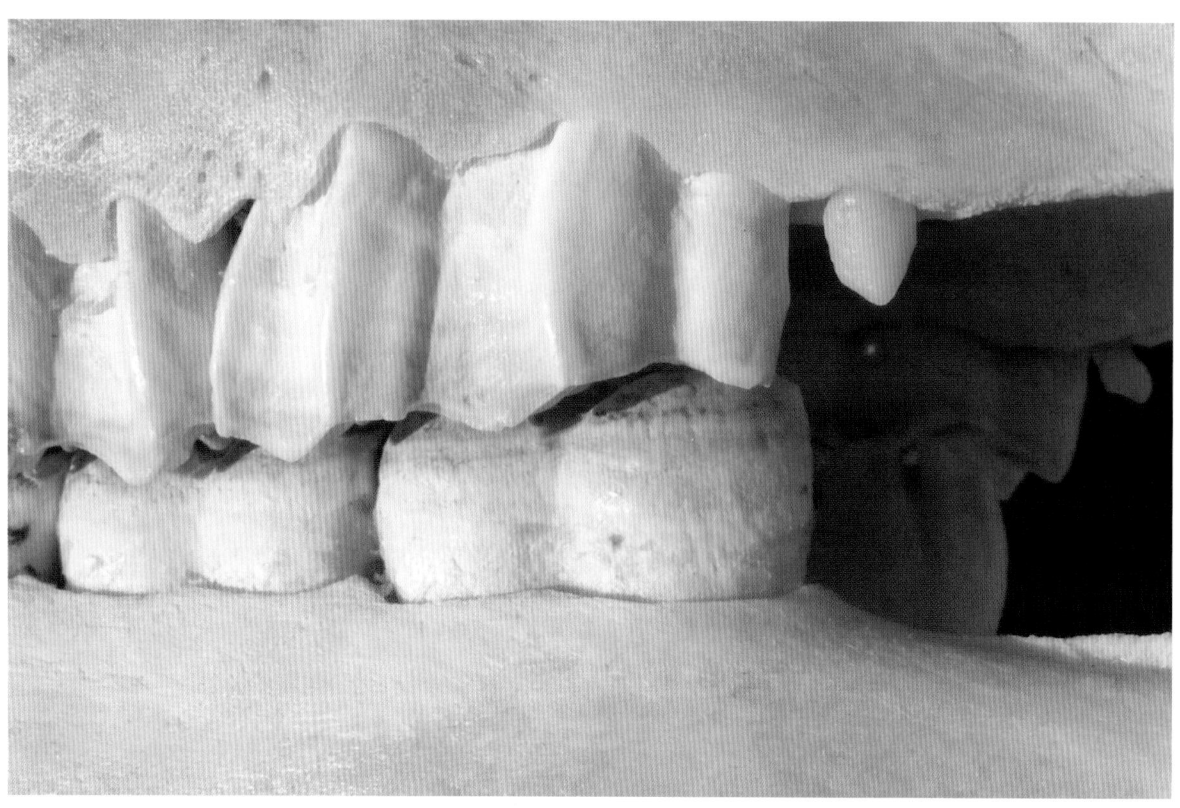

Top:
A normal wolf tooth that is vertical and implanted just in front of the first upper molar.

Below:
On examination, a wolf tooth is clearly visible in front of the first molar.

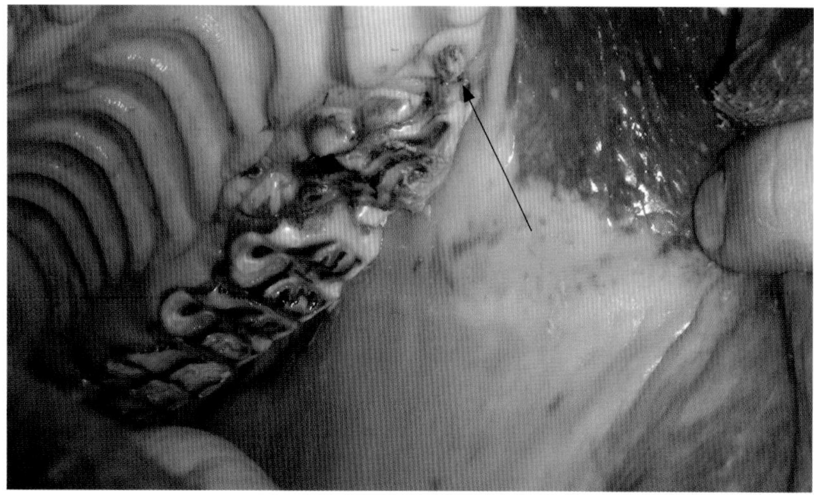

on the front of the first molar: these are much bigger and more robust. Bit pressure on this huge molar does not affect its stability in any way. The tapping of the bit on the wolf teeth can apparently annoy a horse: see how it feels when you tap a metal spoon against your own teeth!

Sometimes the wolf teeth are very sharply pointed so, with pressure from the bit or the noseband, the inside of the cheeks may get hurt. In order to prevent such problems the wolf teeth of young horses are often removed as a preventive measure.

A "blind" wolf tooth in the upper jaw is usually a couple of centimeters in front of the first molar and is implanted obliquely forward. In this

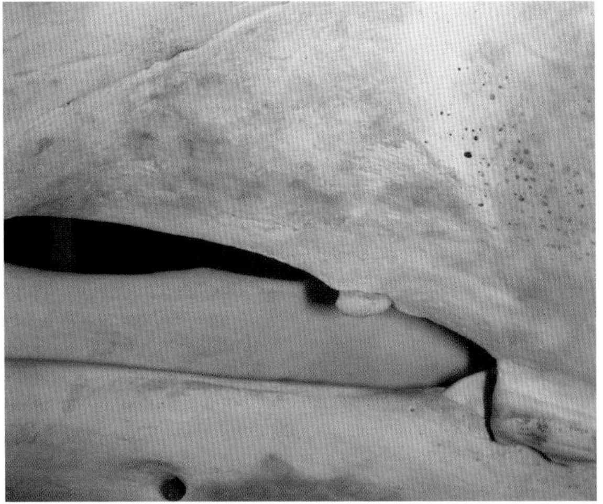

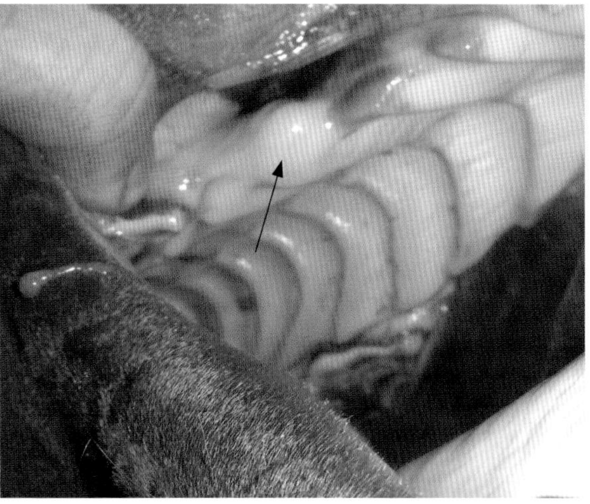

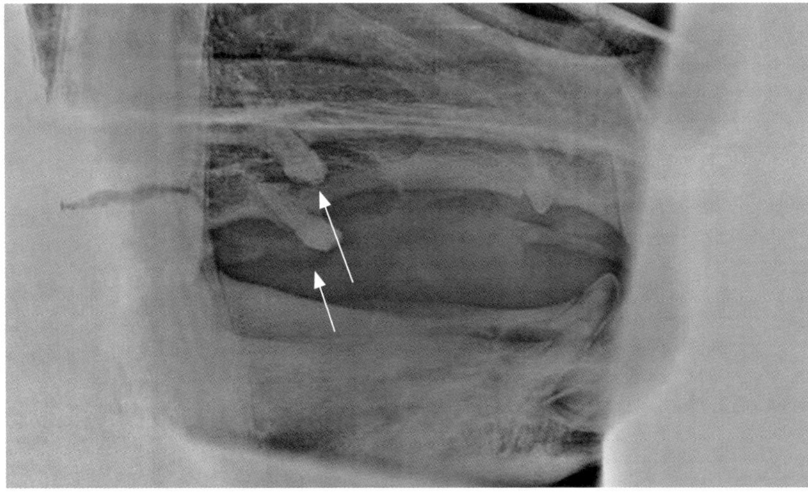

Top left:
A "blind" wolf tooth implanted obliquely forward a few centimeters in front of the first molar.

Top right:
The top of the tooth rarely erupts through the gums because of this angled implantation. So the blind wolf tooth is only visible as a bump on the edge of the hard palate. It can be easily felt through the gum.

Below:
When in doubt, an X-ray of blind wolf teeth can show their position. Two blind wolf teeth can be seen in front of the first molars of this horse.

way, the crown seldom erupts through the gums and can only be felt as a bump at the lower edge of the hard palate. The bit lies precisely at this place against the bars. Thus sometimes the gums covering the bars can be bruised between the bit and the blind wolf tooth: it would be best to remove it. Extracting a wolf tooth or a blind wolf tooth can be performed while the horse is standing up.

Damage to the Bars

Damage to the bars is always caused by too hard of an impact of the bit on the vulnerable bars, and it is nearly always the curb bit that is responsible. The bars consist of a thin layer of soft tissue of only a few millimeters covering the underlying bone of the lower jaw. The leverage of the curb bit in conjunction with the chin groove curb chain sometimes puts enormous pressure on the bars. When there is too much pressure, the gums can be damaged and there can be swelling of the gums of a centimeter thick—with open wounds. Sometimes, we even see that the

Top:
Whenever the bars of a horse are injured by the bit, we talk of "damage to the bars."

Middle:
Injuries can be seen here on the gums of the bars that have been caused by the action of the bit. This is often seen in horses that are ridden with a curb bit and curb chain.

Below:
Sometimes swelling of a centimeter thick can arise on the injured gums from bit pressure. Just think what it is like the next day when the bit is put in the mouth again!

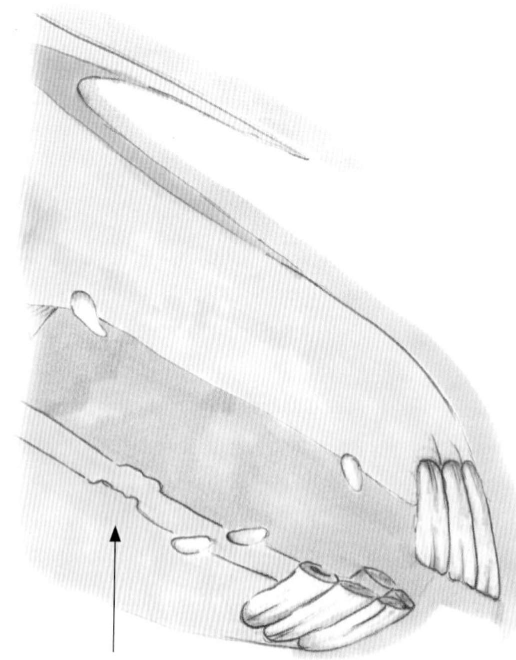

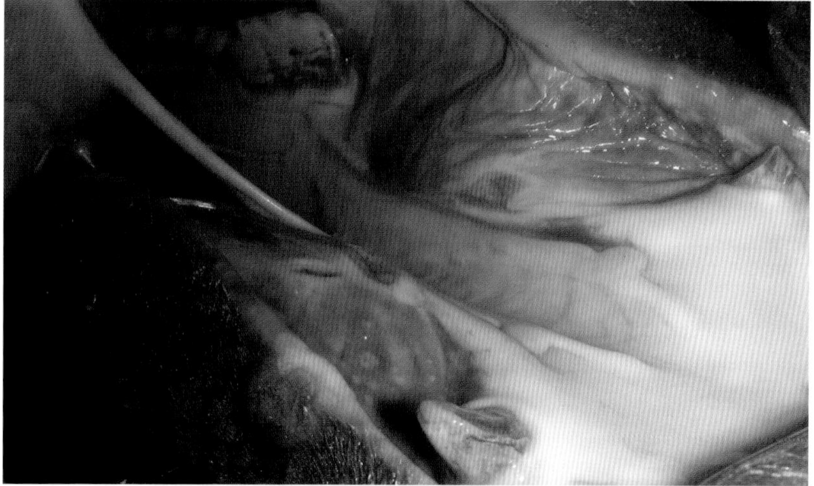

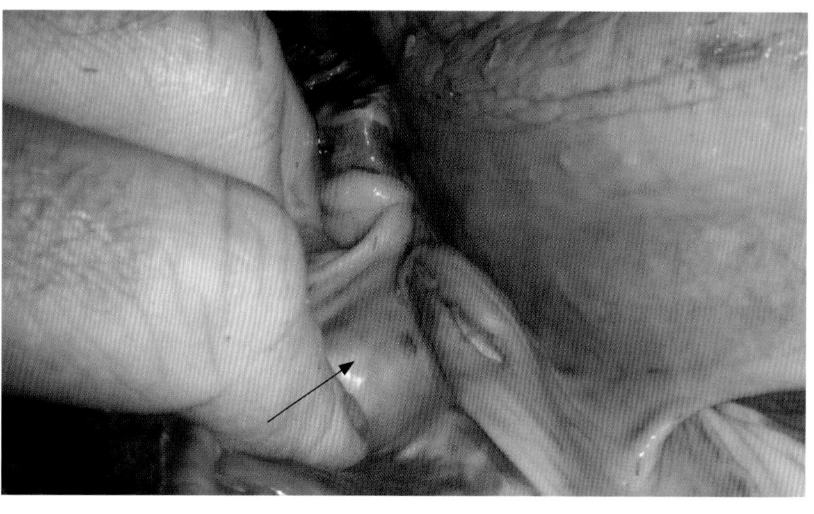

pressure has been so great causing the underlying bone to die off and a bone fragment appear through the gum surface. This is enormously painful for the majority of horses: there is then no way that a horse can be properly ridden on the a bit. Sometimes these horses display blood-flecked foam in the mouth and display a lot of resistance when ridden.

With pressure such as this, some horses have an infection of the bone membrane, which results in new bone production. This causes the upper surface of the jaw bone to become irregular and the covering gum becomes even more bruised by the bit. Very occasionally this bone growth is removed.

Leaving your curb bit hanging in the cupboard for a time is the only way to allow damage to the bars to heal. In the long term, adjusting your way of riding would also be a good idea.

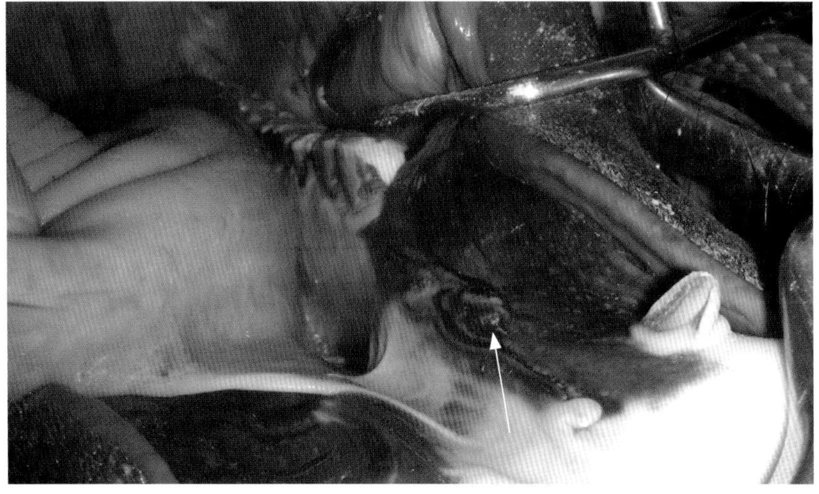

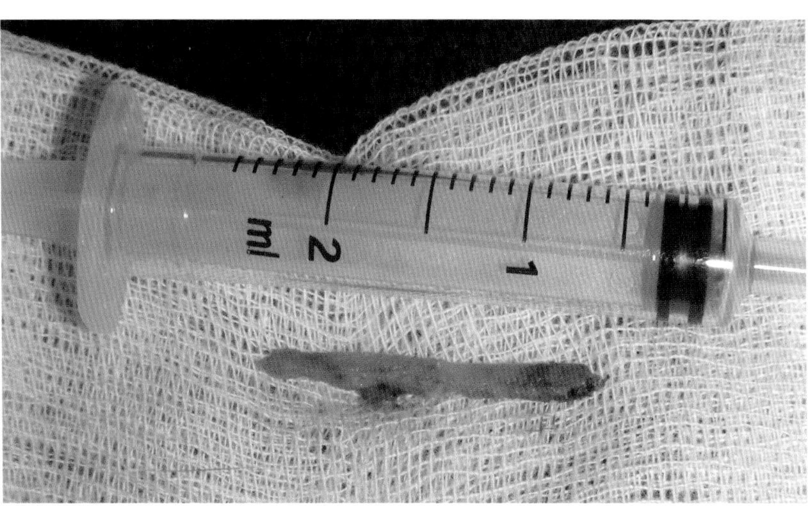

Top:
Damage to the bars of a driving horse that was "difficult" in the mouth. On closer examination, there appeared to be a piece of bone in the first wound; it was removed with forceps. The pressure of the bit had caused a piece of bone to die off and this was ejected as a bone splinter. A horse in this state can best recover by being rested for a few weeks while the bars heal.

Below:
A bone splinter.

CHAPTER II

Disorders of the Molars

The whole structure of the mouth works to create an optimal digestion process. Small defects on tooth surfaces can thoroughly disturb this efficiency. Due to continual eruption of the teeth (the "reserve" crowns emerging from the root), any small irregularities become steadily worse. The key word here, therefore, is prevention. Neglect of the teeth can cause a number of the following disorders at the same time.

The close-fitting molars in each half of the jaw can be seen as one functional whole. The molars fit nicely together and the surface of each arcade of molars is generally level but with small orderly irregularities on the chewing surface. The arcade of teeth is often slightly raised towards the back. If there is abnormal wear somewhere along the grinding plateau, this level plateau becomes unbalanced, and chewing problems or problems with the bit can arise. The following defects are frequently seen.

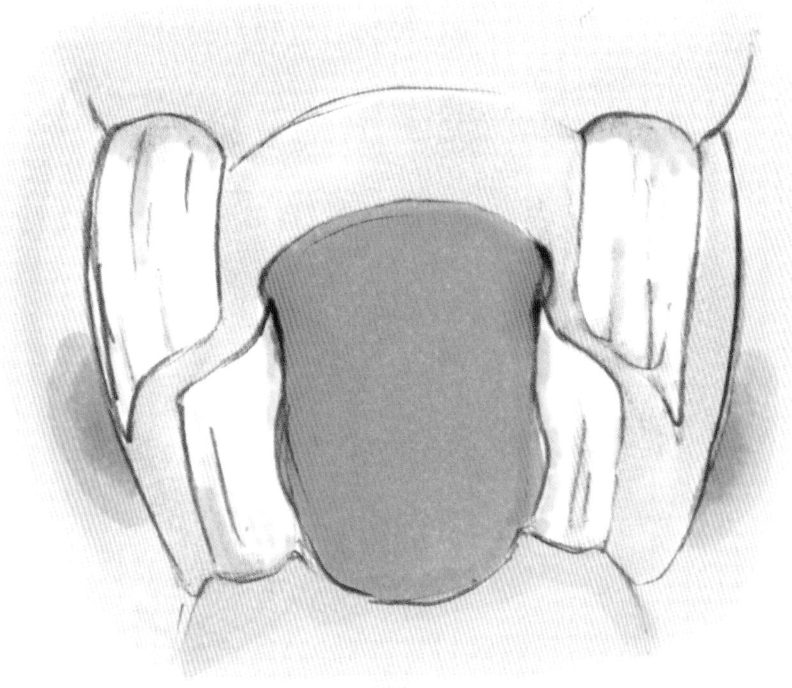

In this cross section of a horse's head at the level of the molars you can see that the upper molars do not meet together evenly with the lower ones: the grinding tables of the upper molars are wider than those of the lower molars, and the tables are not horizontally matched but are, instead, at an oblique angle of about 15 degrees. It is these factors that often cause the development of sharp enamel points on the outside of the upper molars, which can cause injury to the inside of the cheek. Fortunately, the sharp enamel points on the inside of the tables on the lower molars seldom cause injury to the tongue.

Enamel Points

These are commonly—but incorrectly—called "hooks." (For "real" hooks, see below). Sharp enamel points can develop on the cheek side of the upper molars and the tongue side of the lower ones. This happens because of a 10 to 25 degree slant of the chewing surface; the position of the upper molars in relation to the lower ones; the sideways grinding movement; and the "undulating" aspect of the enamel on the outside of the molars. Fodder intake is placed between the molars by the muscles in the tongue and the cheeks and this means there is a close contact between the molars and the cheek or tongue. The sharpness of these enamel points varies greatly between individuals: in some horses they are not too bad, yet in others, they can be razor sharp. The more the upper molars undulate on the outside, the sharper the points usually are.

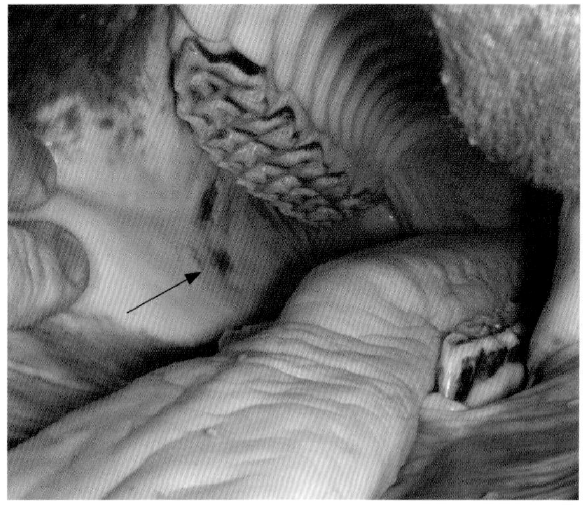

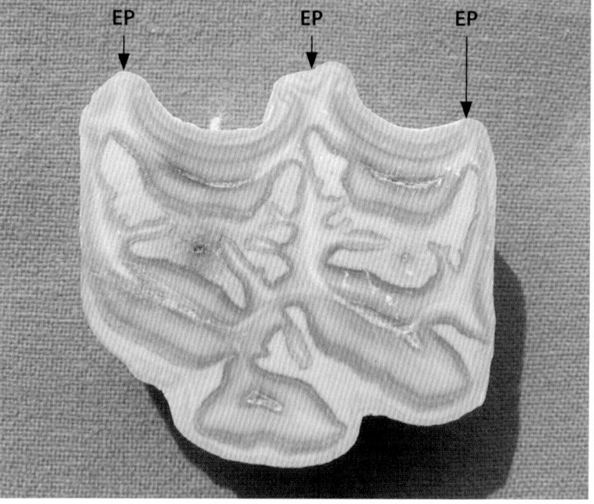

Left and right:
The pronounced undulations on the outside of the molars make the sharp enamel points press against the cheek. These sharp enamel points (EP) can cause considerable damage.

These enamel points often push into the cheek and lead to injury and lesions, which can vary from superficial irritation to a hardened patch of gum with a wound of several millimeters in its center. In some horses there can be injuries along the whole length of the arcade of teeth. Enamel points are present to a certain degree in all horses whose teeth have not been filed within the past six to 12 months. Wounds on the tongue caused by sharp enamel points on the inner side of the lower molars are not seen very often.

A horse can adopt a different chewing pattern to escape pain in the cheeks or tongue, and due to this more limited sideways chewing movement, the sides of the molars receive less abrasion and thus a vicious circle is set up.

Cheek injuries also cause problems in riding and driving horses. The bit rings and high noseband press the insides of the cheeks hard against the enamel points of the upper molars. When the horse tries to relieve the pressure on the cheeks with an abnormal movement of the mouth, most riders have the tendency to tighten the noseband even more. The

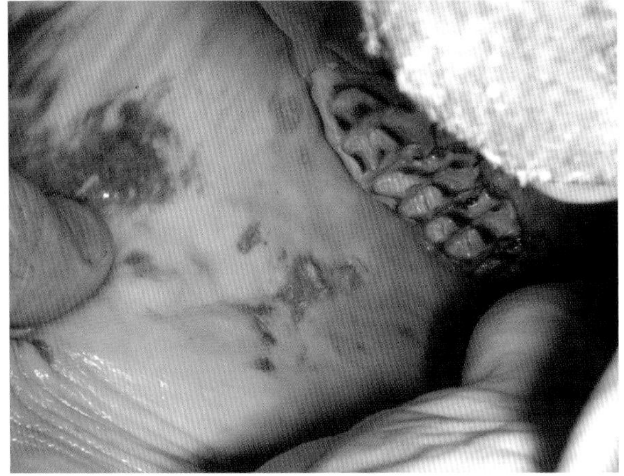

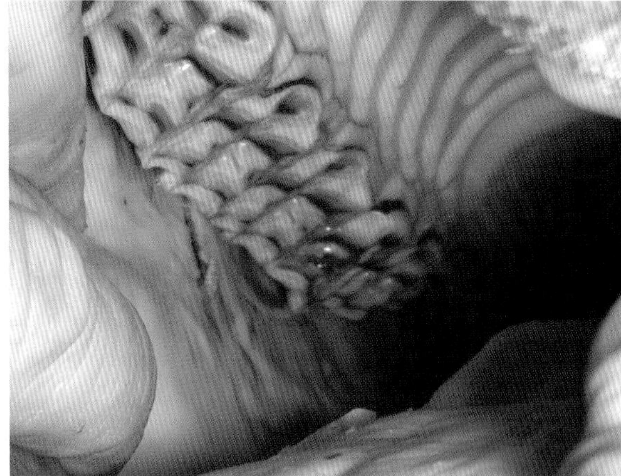

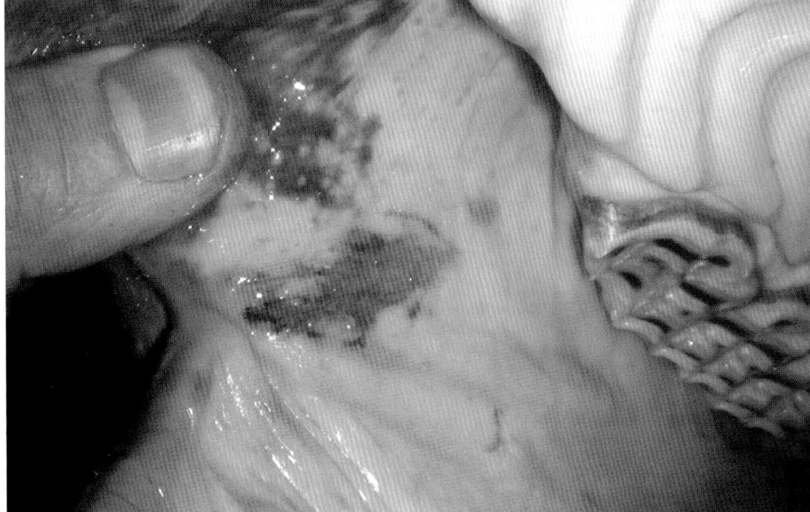

Top left and right:
Injuries seen on the inside of the cheek vary from superficially irritated spots to several small wounds to really deep linear cuts. Sometimes the injured area can be quite large.

Below:
The cheek is pressed against the enamel points of the first molar by pressure from the bit and a tight noseband; this can cause extensive wounds in the horse's cheek and be very uncomfortable.

horse then resists even more when it feels the pressure of the enamel points. If the noseband is loosened by a couple of notches instead of being tightened and you notice that the horse is quieter in its mouth, then both you and your horse will, in all likelihood, benefit from some equine dental treatment.

The floating of these enamel points is the basis of a routine treatment when a horse is being worked. As long ago as 1906, Dr. Merillat said, "Cutting and floating enamel points is the principal work of the animal dentist." We often notice that the outer side of the two farthest back upper molars are neglected as these are difficult to reach in a horse not under anesthetic.

Can these tiny enamel points really cause so much suffering? Just imagine something pricking the inside of your cheek; you would probably make an appointment with the dentist or doctor as soon as possible. We expect horses to perform concentrated work for half an hour to an hour and react to our rein aids. Many, many horses in these circumstances are distracted by one or more enamel points pricking the insides of their cheeks.

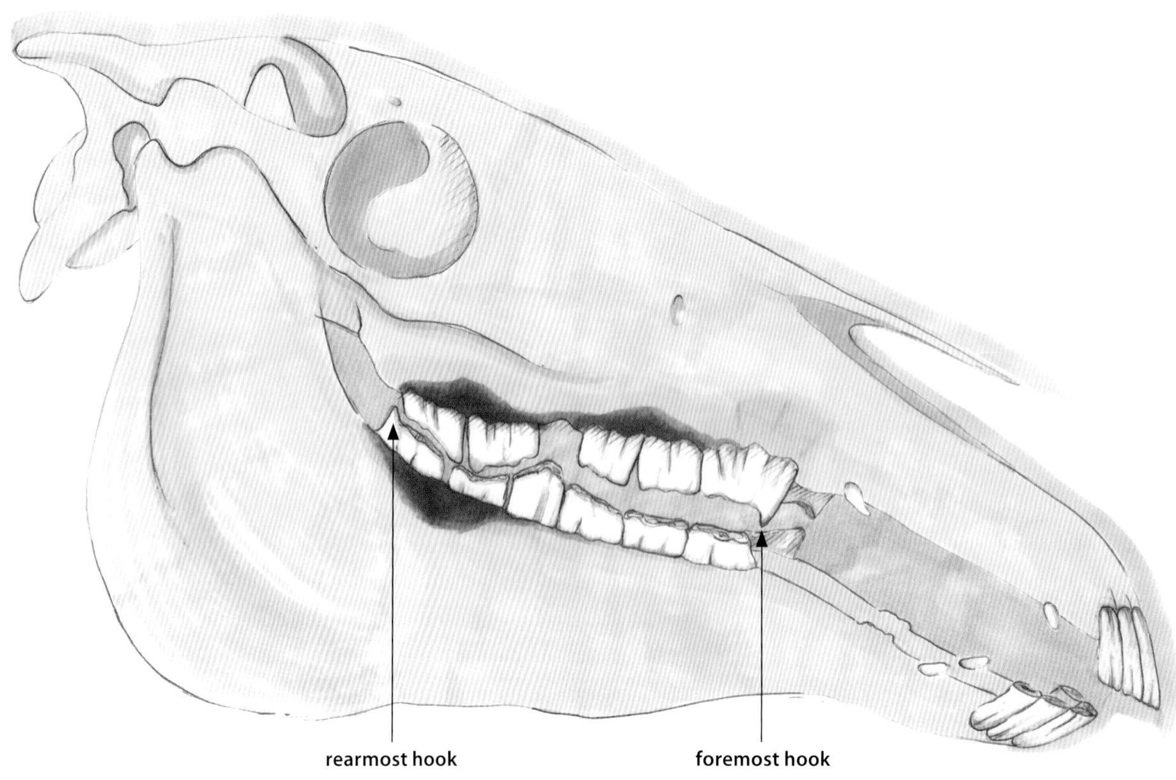

A foremost or rearmost hook is developed due to lack of abrasion in front of the first molar and lack of abrasion at the back of the last molar.

Foremost and Rearmost Hooks

In contrast to the enamel points these are "real" hooks. These often appear on the front of the first upper molar (106 and 206) and at the back of the last lower molar (311 and 411). The table of the molar concerned lies slightly beyond the table of the opposing molar thus a part of the table is no longer worn down and a pointed elevation develops on part of the table: a hook. The more easily observed foremost hook often goes hand in hand with a rear hook, which is difficult to see. Some of these hooks can be rather sharp and cause cheek injuries or lesions in the gums opposite.

The foremost or rearmost hook can also be the cause of problems with riding on the bit. When a horse is going well on the bit, it relaxes the lower jaw, which is lightly pushed forward. When the mouth is closed, big hooks will restrict the forward and backward movement of the lower jaw. This causes abnormal pressure and pain in the jaw joint that in turn, may cause the horse to no longer bend its head very well.

The hooks not only have to be rounded off but should also be levelled to the normal grinding plateau. This is easily achieved with the foremost hook because of its position in the mouth, but rather more difficult to achieve with the rearmost hook.

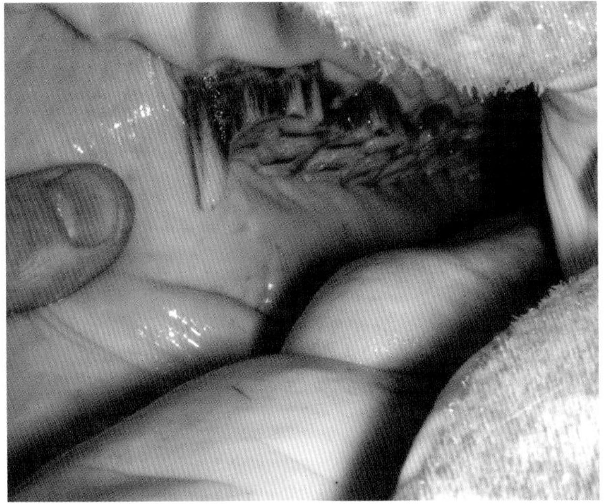
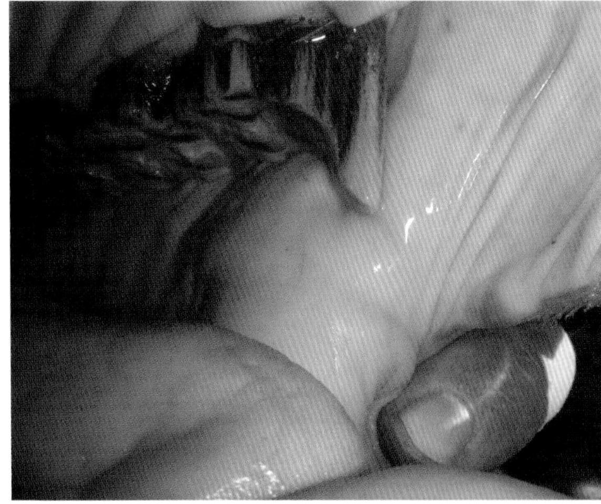
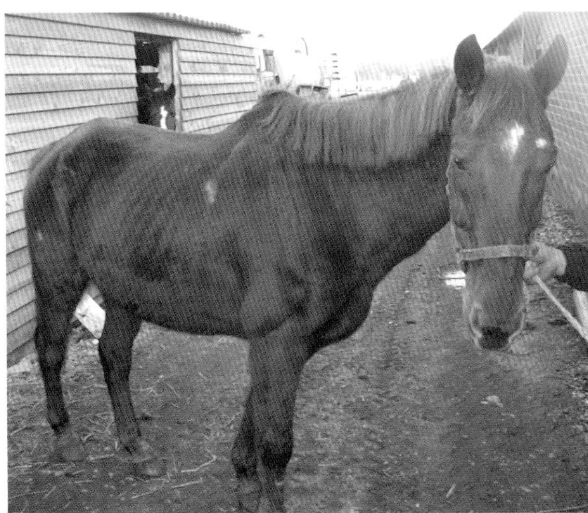
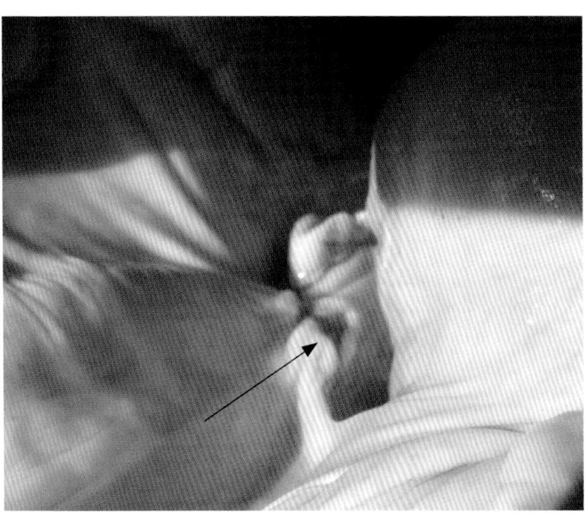
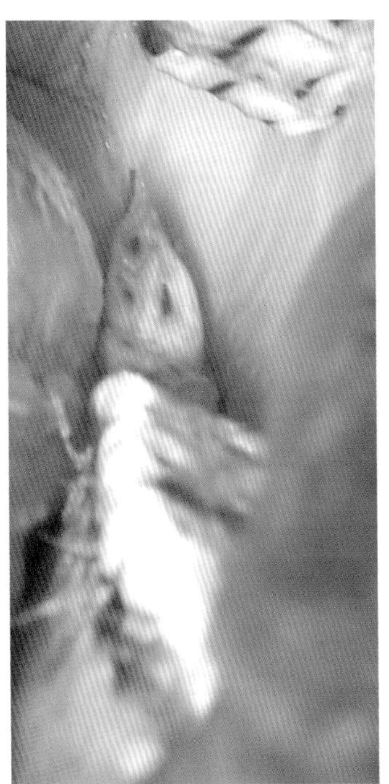
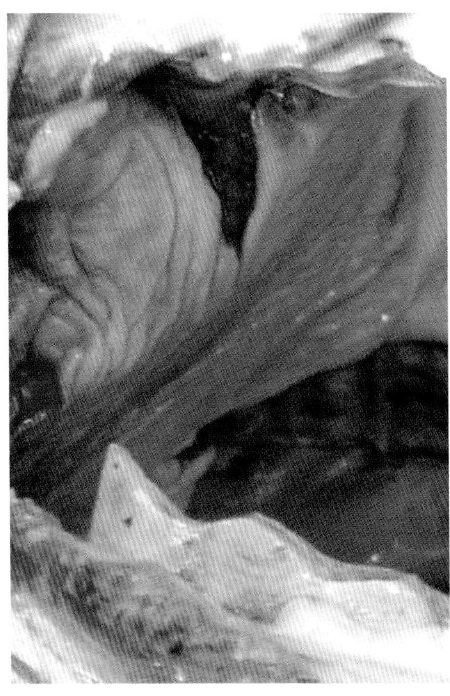

Top four pictures:
The horse shown had extremely long hooks on both first upper molars. It fed poorly, dropped wads of compacted forage from its mouth and had lost a great deal of weight. The hooks were so long that the pointed ends pressed into the bars just in front of the first lower molar. With each grinding action this horse bit into its own bars.

Below left:
The last lower molar clearly rises in a sharp point at the back. This is called the rearmost hook.

Below right:
Although this rear hook (411) is only half a centimeter high, it was the cause of a cut in the palate opposite.

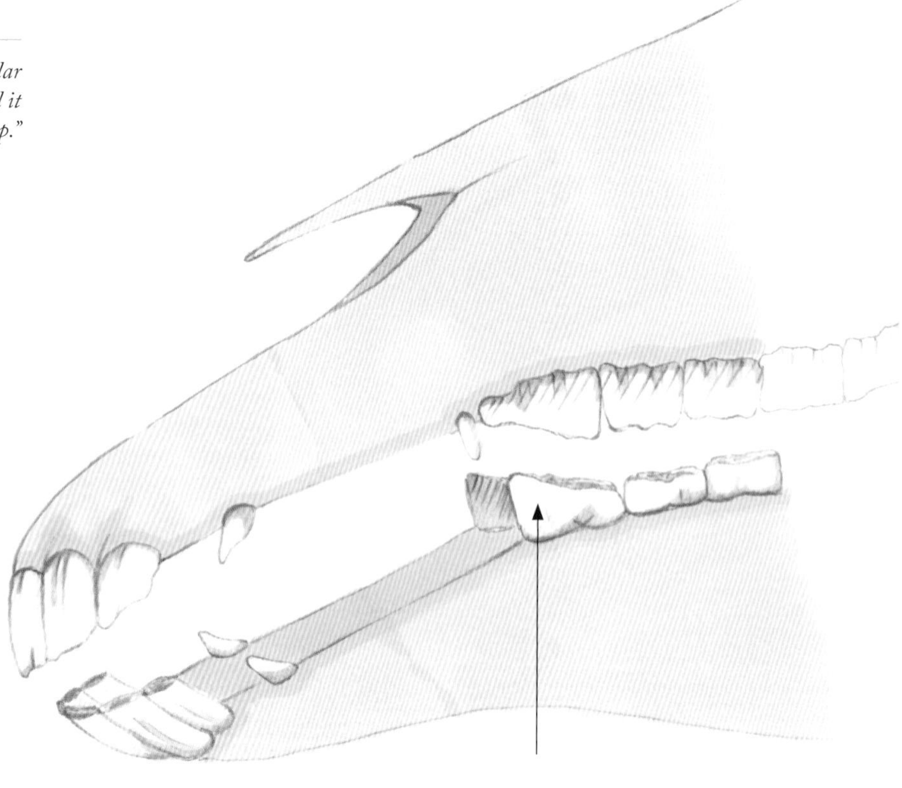

When the whole table of a molar slants up at one side, we call it a "ramp."

Ramps

In contrast to a hook, in a "ramp" we see a gradual "rising" of the table of a molar from the front to the back, or vice versa. Here, the whole table is involved whereas in the case of a hook, only part of the table of a molar is higher. We see ramps mostly in the first and the last molar of the lower jaw. At the same time, the table of the opposite molar will be more worn down.

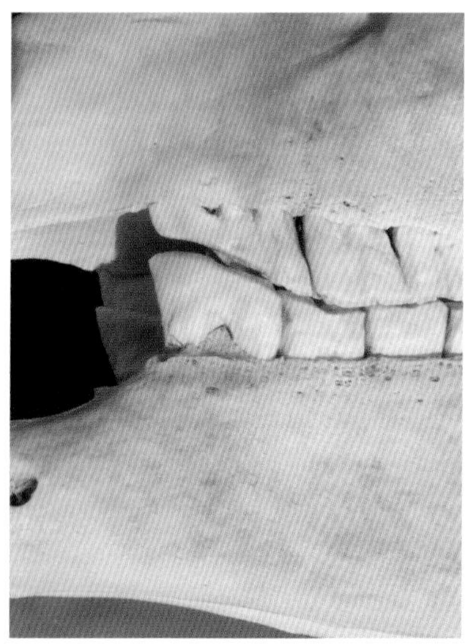

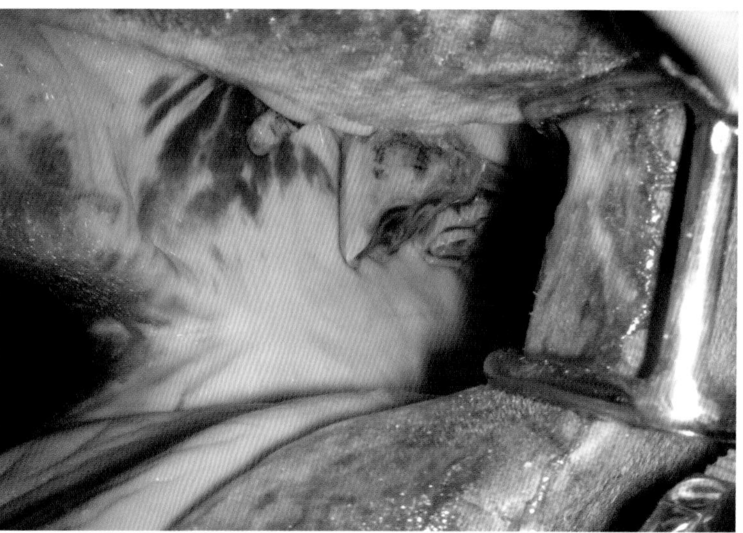

Below left: The table of the first molar is clearly inclined upward at the front of the tooth, which causes the table of the opposite tooth to be excessively worn away.

Below right: The first molar (106) of this horse is a ramp. Note also the wolf tooth that is implanted far forward. This wolf tooth constantly touches the bit.

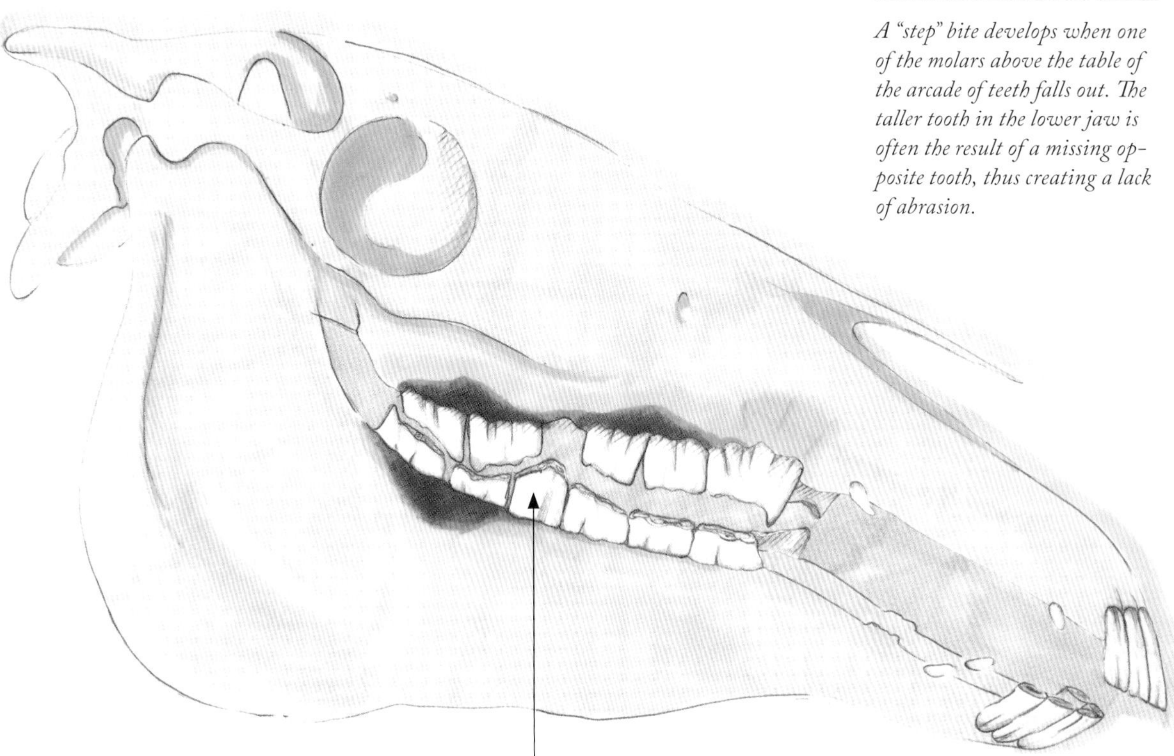

A "step" bite develops when one of the molars above the table of the arcade of teeth falls out. The taller tooth in the lower jaw is often the result of a missing opposite tooth, thus creating a lack of abrasion.

"Step" Mouth

Step teeth arise when there is no abrasion or little abrasion on the table of a molar. This is mostly seen when the opposing tooth has been lost, and as abrasion is absent, the molar grows up into the empty space. It rises clearly above the normal grinding plateau and can distinctly upset the chewing movement. Due to the tooth loss, there is also more room in the arcade of teeth, so the teeth stand a little apart from each other. These horses definitely need an annual dental correction.

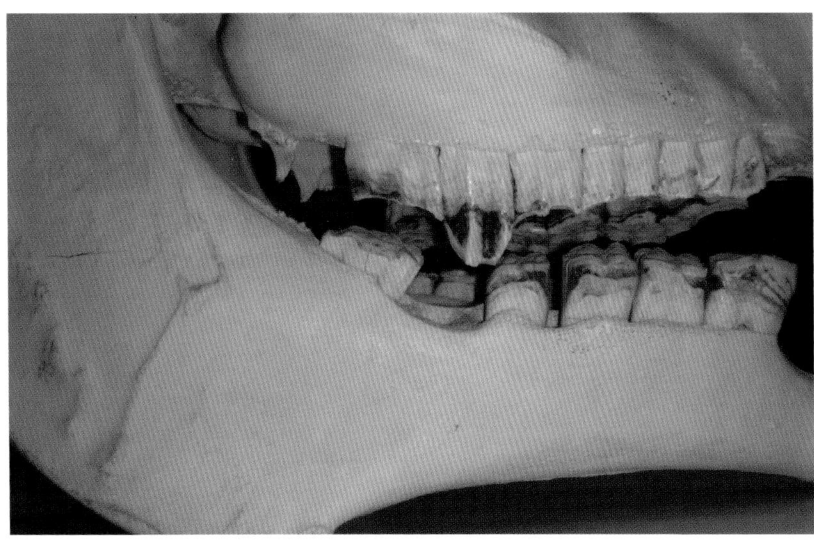

Due to a missing tooth (410), the opposite tooth (110) has not been worn down anymore, and consequently, it has grown down into the opening that's been created. These step teeth seriously hinder the horse's chewing mechanism.

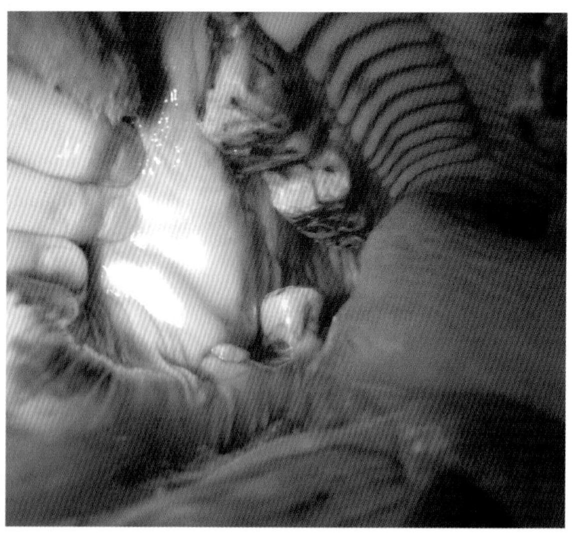

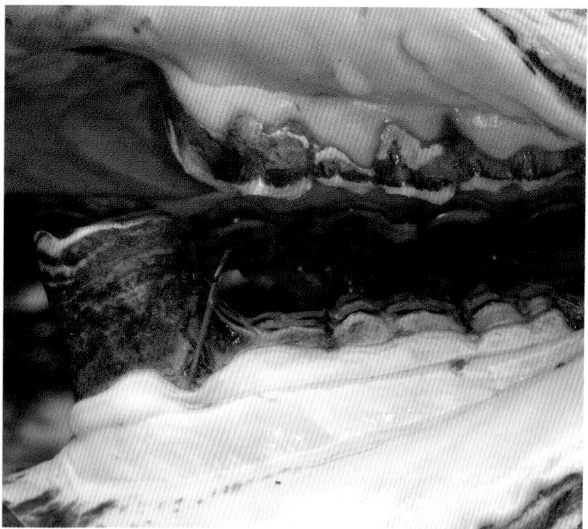

Above left: In this horse of 26 years, most of the lower molars have been worn down to the gums except the third molar (408). The erosion of the opposite tooth (108) was clearly the cause of a step bite here.

Top right: Step mouth. The first molar (306) here is nearly four centimeters higher than the table of the lower arcade of teeth. The opposite tooth has been worn away deep into the gums. Actually, this horse should have been treated 10 years ago.

"Wave" Mouth

This is an up-and-down curving in the arcade of teeth, often where several teeth are involved. There is usually some other defect in the mouth that is the base cause of the problem. The horse adopts a defective chewing cycle, which worsens if the set of teeth is not treated. Due to the level of the dental defect and because several teeth are involved, a correction of a wave mouth can often not be treated in one session. For example, if we reduce the height of a curve with four teeth to the correct table level, an opening is created between these and the four opposing molars and the horse loses a great percentage of its chewing surface.

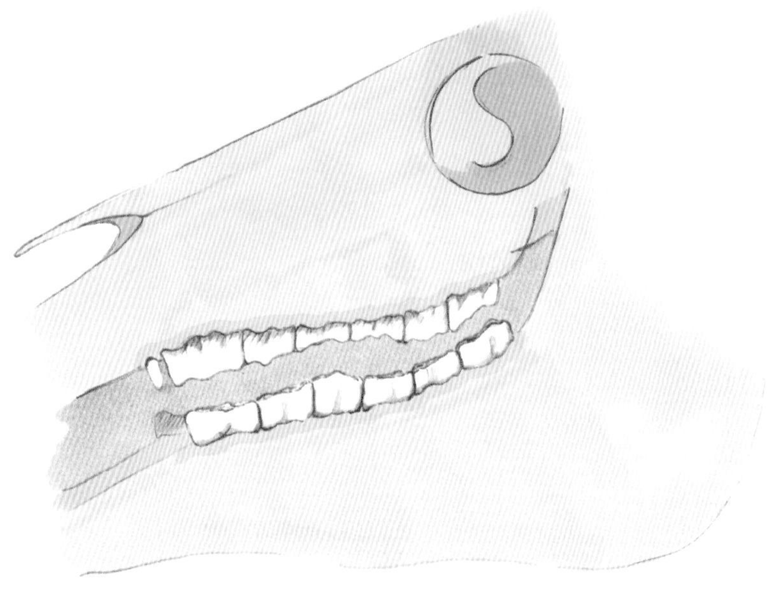

When the teeth in an arcade rise and fall, we call it a "wave" bite.

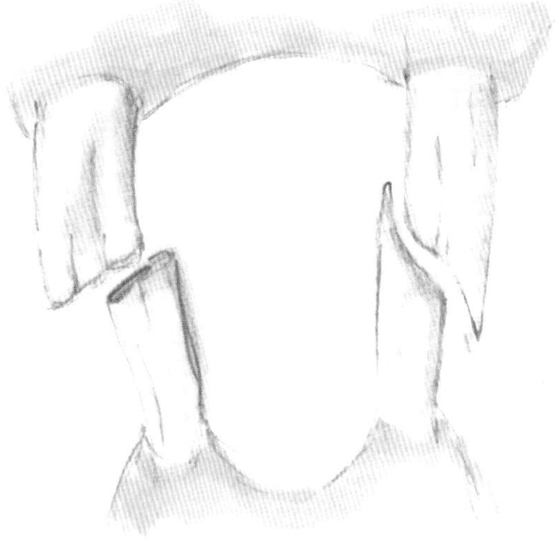

Whenever the slope between the table of the lower and upper molars is greater than 35 degrees, it's called a "shear" bite. It hinders the normal sideways-chewing movement.

"Shear" Mouth

In the case of shear teeth, the angle of the tables of the upper and lower molars is far greater than 25 degrees: this angle can even be as much as 50 or 60 degrees. With teeth such as these, a sideways-grinding movement is impossible, and the angle of the tables only becomes greater by abnormal abrasion. Shear teeth are usually only seen on one side of the mouth. It is caused by a painful process whereby the animal has adopted an abnormal chewing pattern. Having shear teeth in both arcades is rarely seen and is caused by a too narrow lower jaw in relation to the upper jaw.

Horses with a shear mouth cannot therefore really grind their food any more but chew it instead—as humans do, which makes it impossible for the horse to reduce roughage suitably. The long sides of the molars are also frequently extremely sharp. This defect cannot usually be corrected in one session. Frequently, there are underlying problems present. An

Below left:
On the far right of this photo is a normal upper molar with a table slope of about 15 degrees. This angle can be as much as 65 degrees as is seen on the shear tooth on the far left. A tooth like this makes sideways-chewing movement practically impossible.

Below right:
This horse has a one-sided shear bite (left side of picture). The slope of the tables is nearly 45 degrees. Notice the clear difference between these teeth and the normal molars on the right side. The blue patch in the back is an artificial plug put into the socket after the removal of the back molar.

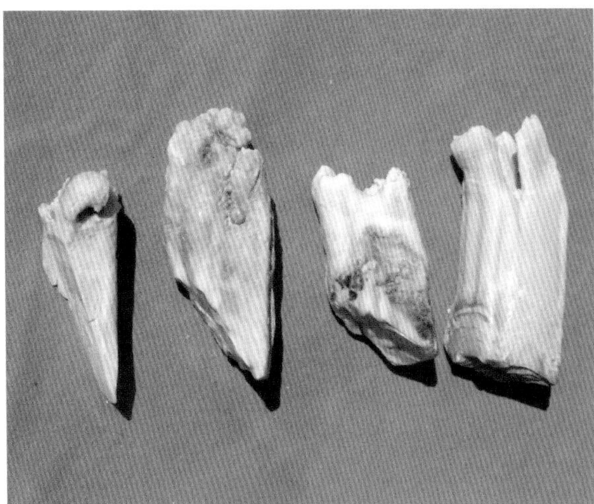

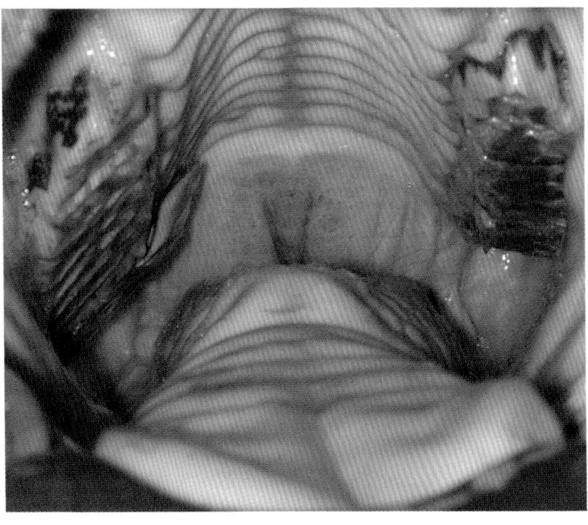

untreated shear mouth leads to eating problems, ensuing weight loss and sometimes even the death of the horse.

When the defect is discovered in time, the situation with the grinding plateau can usually be completely rectified. If you wait until your horse can barely eat anymore and it has already suffered great weight loss, then you are usually five or 10 years too late for regaining a full recovery.

Top illustration: The remains of the milk teeth that are situated on the future tables of the permanent molars are called "caps."

Below left: In this view of the teeth sockets of a two-year-old, you can see the permanent teeth above the caps. Notice the long sharp "projections" at the root ends of these caps. These can prick the gums when the caps become loose.

Below right: In this cross section of a horse's head you see the remains of the milk teeth: the caps. The permanent teeth are ready to erupt into the mouth when the caps fall out.

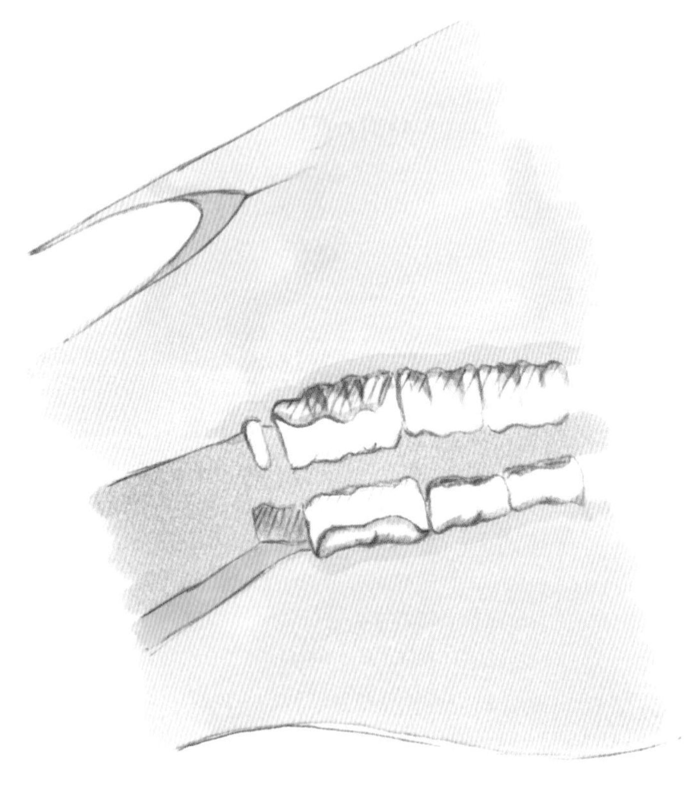

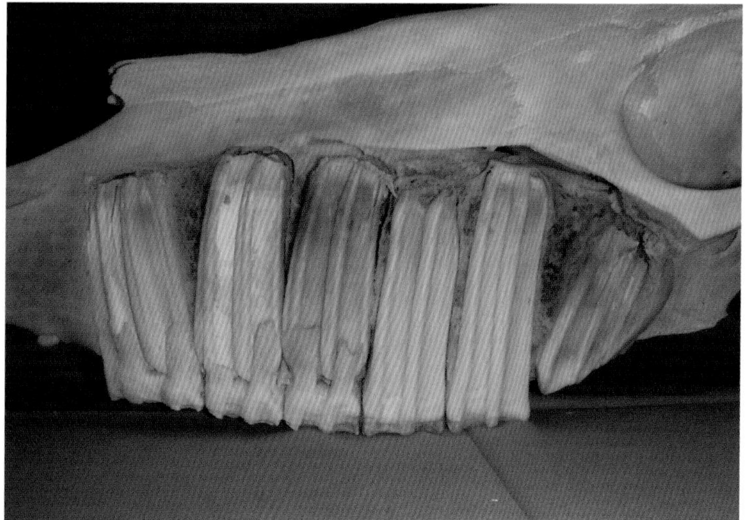

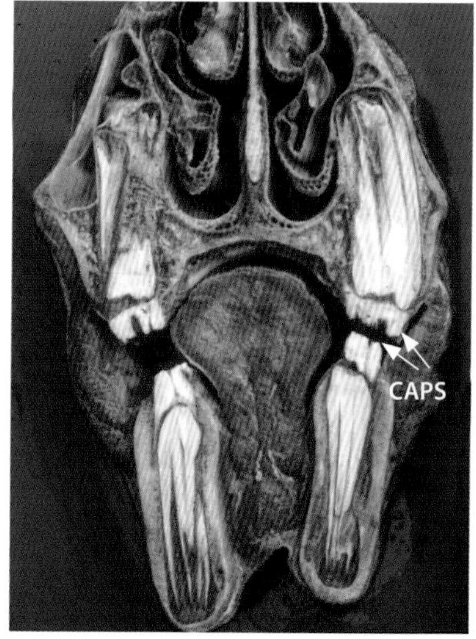

Caps

Caps are the remains of the first three milk molars that get pushed out by the eruption of the underlying permanent molars. They are usually flat rectangular slivers with, on each side, two sharp peaks: the remains of the former root. These can be extremely sharp and when the cap has partly come loose it can prick into the surrounding gum. If a horse—in the teeth-replacement stage—suddenly displays problems with chewing, this could be one of the causes.

Sometimes there is a persistent cap on the third molar. This is then caught in between the permanent second and third molars. The force of the upward growth of the third permanent molar underneath is sometimes not strong enough to eject the cap into the mouth. This cap must, then, be removed.

The caps can be easily removed with a caps forceps. If the caps are removed too soon, it can cause damage to the underlying permanent molar.

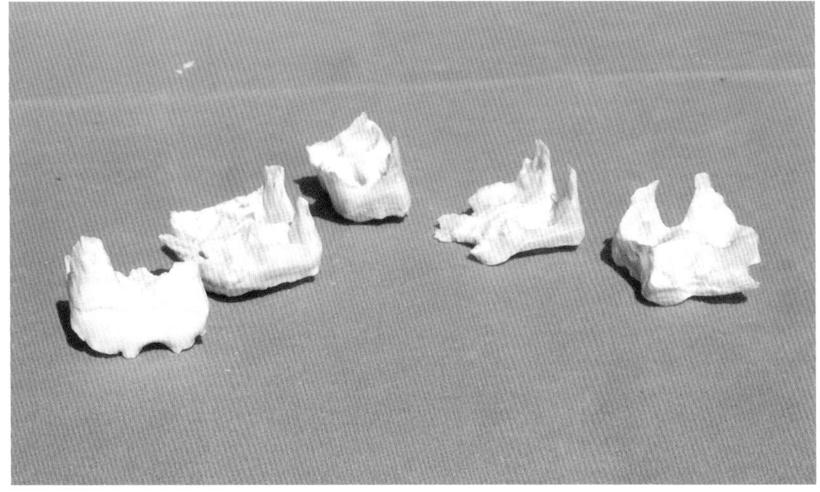

Top:
The long "ends" of the remains of the roots can be clearly seen on these caps. When caps are only loosely attached to the permanent teeth, these bits sticking out prick into the surrounding gums.

Below left and right:
A clear division between the cap and the permanent teeth can be observed in the skull (left) and in the living horse (right). This cap can be removed.

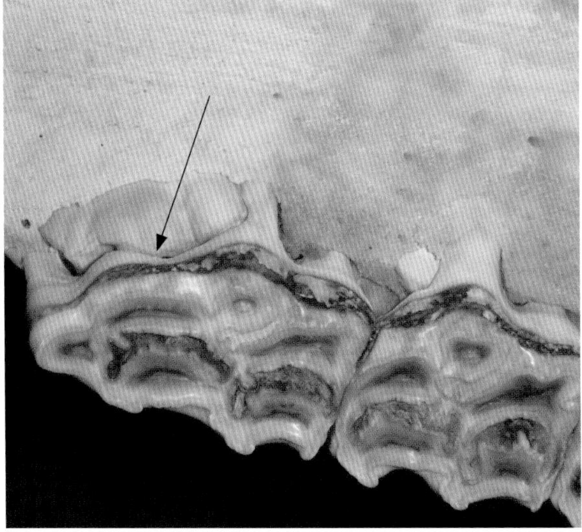

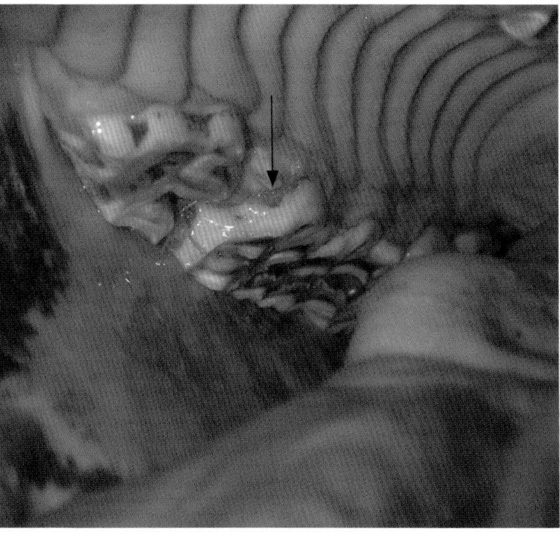

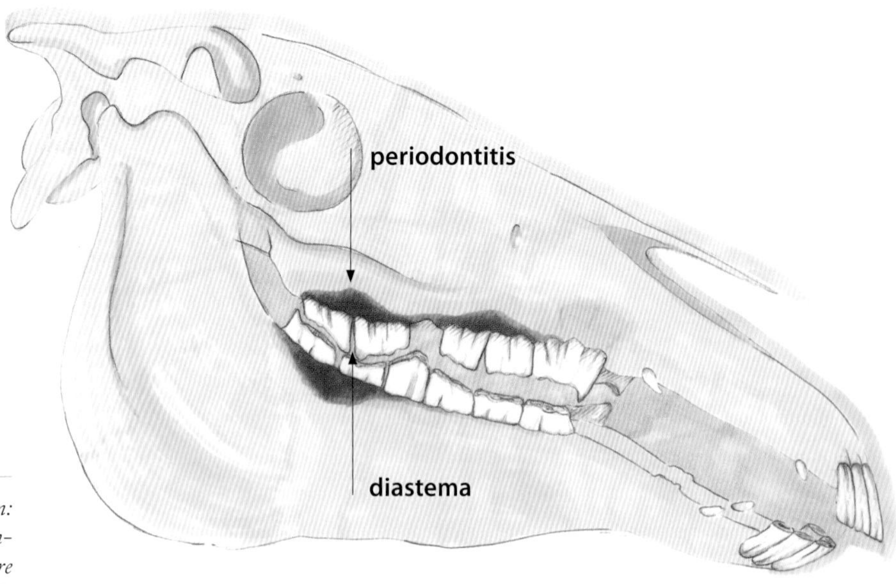

Top, illustration: A diastema is a split-like opening between two molars where food can become wedged. This can cause periodontitis.

Below left: Shown here is how grass can get wedged in the diastemas. This can cause periodontitis, an inflammation of the surrounding tissue, which can be extremely painful.

Below right: As the mouth is being closed, the foremost hook always makes the first molar push forward. This created a diastema between the first and second molars, which resulted in the development of periodontitis. Regular floating of the front of the upper molars could have prevented all this.

It is only wise to remove a cap when it is already loose and there is a clear line of division visible between the cap and the permanent tooth.

Diastema and Periodontitis

A diastema is the narrow opening between two molars that, normally speaking, should be neatly fitted together. This situation is usually prevented by the backward-facing position of the first molar and the forward position of the fifth and sixth molars. Normally, due to the pressure from both ends of the arcade of teeth, the molars are neatly close-fitting and they can function as a whole.

An insufficiently oblique-angled position of the first or the last two molars can mean there is not enough of this pressure, and this can cause an opening between the molars. The molars also narrow down towards

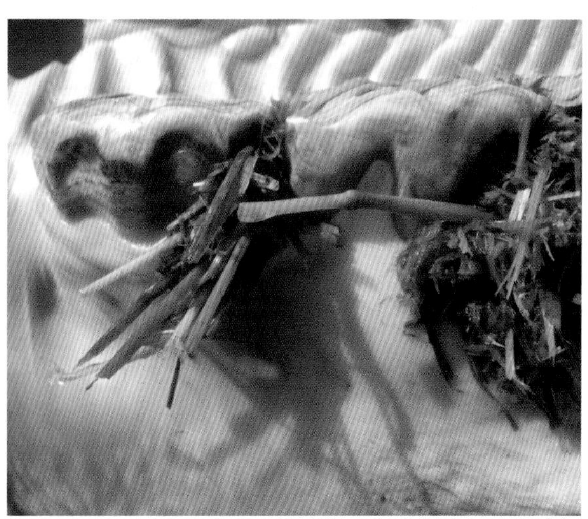

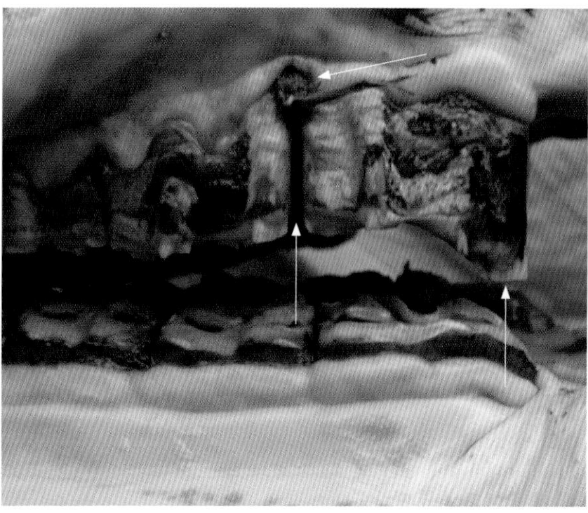

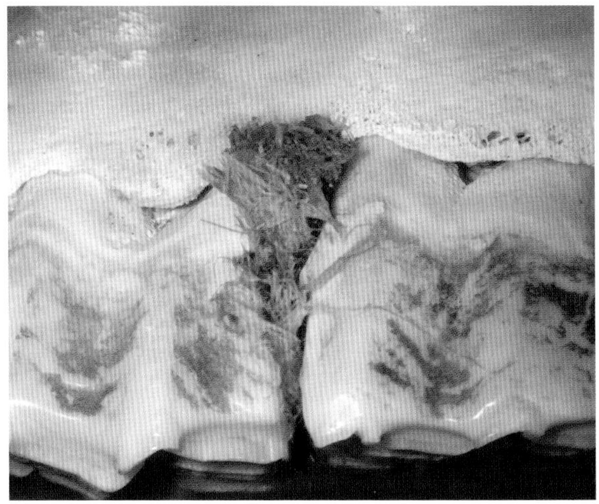

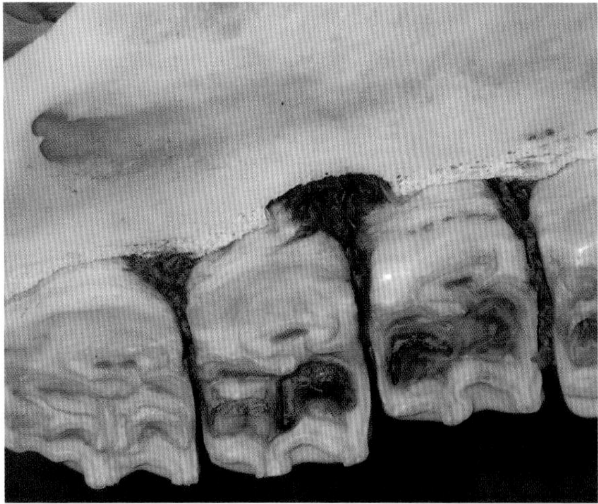

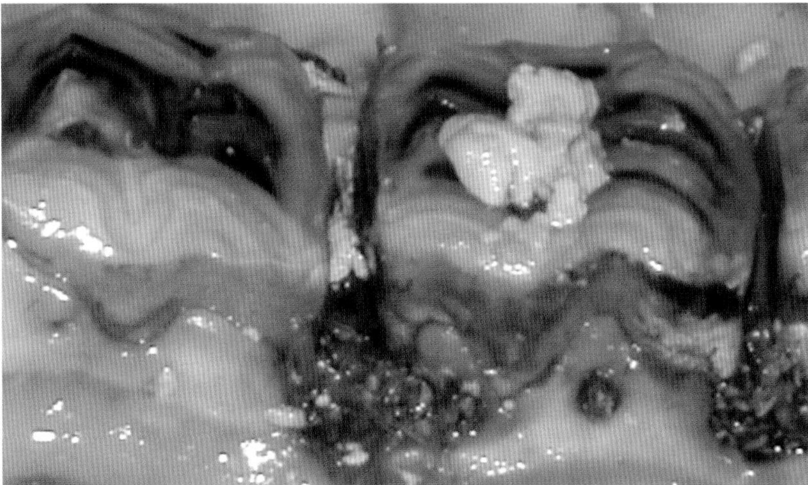

Top left:
A diastema is often built up like a valve. The opening at the table end is narrower than the space above: food gets pushed up but cannot get out.

Top right:
Sometimes food is "pushed" several centimeters deep between the teeth so that perionditis is extensive with the entire surrounding root socket affected.

Below:
This 24-year-old horse had to be put down because of sinusitis caused by extensive diastemas and periodontitis. The horse displayed a chronic suppurating, runny left nostril. When the diastemas between the last three molars were rinsed out, clumps of pus were washed out into the mouth.

the root. This can therefore, in the older horse, be partly responsible for the development of diastemas. Abnormal pressure on the tables—such as in a step mouth or wave mouth—can also cause the teeth to be pushed apart. Food can then be forced up between the teeth while the horse is chewing.

If the opening at the table end of the molar is narrower than it is at the gum end, you will see mostly rough stalks of forage caught between the teeth. Compare this to a piece of apple or meat that gets stuck in between your teeth at the level of the gums; you can then deal with this by flossing or using a toothpick to rid yourself of the irritant. Horses cannot usually remove the food stuck between their teeth with their tongues and thus they suffer continuous discomfort and pain in the gums underneath.

In addition, food stuck between the teeth creates a perfect environment for bacteria to multiply. This then causes inflammation at the edge of the gum that can affect the outside of the tooth: now we talk of periodontitis.

Periodontitis is a painful condition that damages the gums, the dental cementum and, at a more advanced stage, the fibers that hold the tooth in the bone and the bony tooth socket. It can eventually result in the tooth loosening completely and falling out. Sometimes, food is pushed down next to the teeth for a couple of centimeters and occasionally, it goes all the way along the tooth into the sinuses. Consequently, it can cause an enormous sinus infection or a pus-filled fistula in the lower jaw.

Diastemas are mostly found in older horses and mostly between the last three lower molars. In the early stages, most diastemas fortunately do not lead to obvious clinical problems. The most obvious issue with diastemas and the accompanying periodontitis is when the horse lets wads of hay or lumps of concentrated feed fall from its mouth, so-called "quidding." This happens because of the pain caused by the extra pressure on the inflamed gums from chewing. During an examination, when pressure is put on the affected gums, the horse usually reacts by pulling its head back. There is also a bad smell from its mouth due to the bacterial fermentation of the food wedged in between the teeth.

When an older horse drops balls or wads of food and continues to do so even after a correction of the grinding plateau, then it is almost certain that there are diastemas with accompanying periodontitis present at the back between the molars. A thorough examination of the mouth with a sufficiently strong light source and a dental mirror is then indicated.

Most horses do not show obvious symptoms. In some, the chronic pain results in change in behavior, or new problems when being ridden.

Sometimes diastemas with periodontitis are found in the young horse going through teeth replacement. The food is often stuck between the temporary milk teeth and the permanent teeth. These horses often display difficulty chewing. When the milk teeth have been replaced, the problem is usually resolved without having to resort to treatment.

Treatment for the diastemas and the underlying periodontitis consists of the removal of the wedged food. This can be done with long forceps or by cleaning the space between the teeth with water and/or air pressure. This is usually only a temporary solution: it's a good idea to exchange the hay or the dry feed for softer grass or grass pellets.

A more permanent solution is to "open out" the diastema up to the level of the table. The opening made between the teeth is usually widened by about 6 mm so that food can no longer become wedged between the teeth. At the same time, we seek to restore a normal grinding plateau by correcting irregularities on the molar tables. In so doing, extreme care is taken to ensure that the table of the tooth opposing the diastema is properly leveled. We often see, because of the gap between the teeth, that a transverse ridge has been created on the opposite table because there has been less abrasion in that place. These ridges then force the food even more firmly into the diastema and are the cause of even more pain.

When the inflammation is not too far advanced, the periodontitis can disappear by removing the cause. In well-advanced periodontitis, though, extraction of the tooth is sometimes unavoidable.

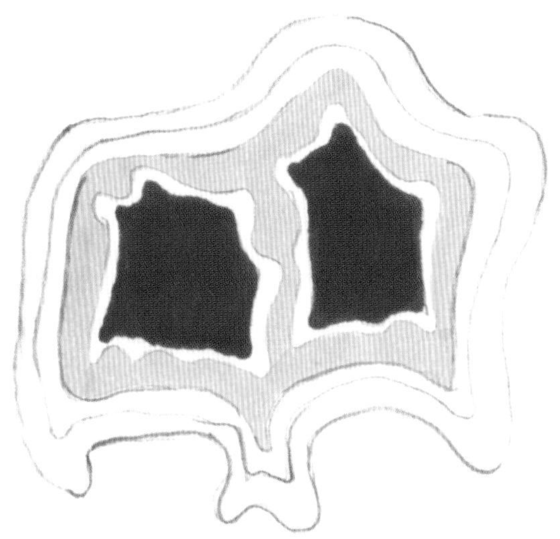

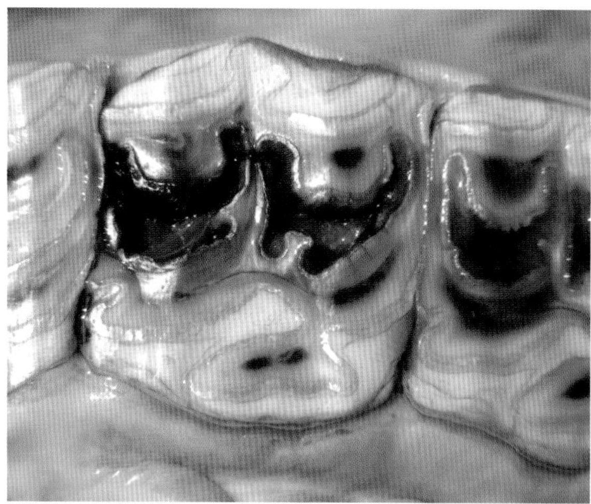

Left:
"Caries" or decay is caused by the fermentation of sugars in the feed by bacteria in the mouth.

Right:
Caries often develops in the two enamel depressions of the fourth and fifth upper molars. It causes pain in horses just as it does in humans. The tooth can even break open from the erosion caused by the decay in its center.

Caries (cavities)

Toothache in humans is, for the greater part, caused by "caries," or cavities. In horses, caries rarely produces clear symptoms.

Caries is a disease caused by the fermentation of sugars in the feed from bacteria in the mouth. This causes a lessening of the degree of acid round the teeth and subsequently there is decalcification of the substance of the teeth: eventually the structure of a tooth is affected and a cavity appears.

Caries in horses is mostly seen in the center of the two enamel "rings" on the table of the fourth and fifth upper molars. Caries is observable by the obvious black color of the affected parts. In a very advanced state, the center of the tooth structure can be so weakened that it breaks in its length down to the root. It is only in this late stage that affected horses display eating problems.

Sometimes caries can be seen affecting the outside of nearly all the molars. This is mostly found in horses that have had feed with a high sugar content, such as molasses; it also arises when they are given cattle feed with added acid.

In the last couple of years, horses have been treated for caries appearing on the tables of their molars – in just the same way humans are. The affected parts are drilled and the cavity is filled. The aim of this treatment is to strengthen the tooth structure and to prevent any possible breakage. Whether this is really worthwhile still has to be determined.

Molar Fractures

When there is a molar fracture it is usually a lengthwise fracture of the upper molars, and mostly involves the fourth and fifth molars. In their center, the upper molars have two enamelled indentations (enamel "rings"

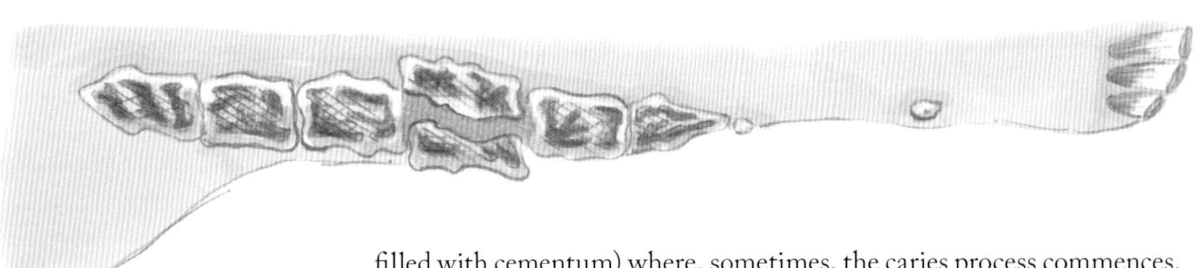

filled with cementum) where, sometimes, the caries process commences. This is bacterial damage of the cement and the underlying enamel layer. This causes the tooth to become hollowed out in the center of the table so that the structure becomes weakened. The chewing of a hard substance can act like a wedge being pushed into this central hollow, which then causes the molar to break in half. The two halves can be further forced apart at the table by food being forced into the hollow during normal chewing. The outside half is often pushed into the cheek, which then causes injury. The inside half is pushed against the hard palate. Feeding problems occur only weeks or months after the original fracture. These problems are then mostly caused by the fact that one of the fragments is so far forced apart by the food being pushed in that it results in an injury in the cheek or tongue.

Top, illustration:
A molar fracture is nearly always a break that runs in the length of the table.

Middle:
A fracture of the second upper molar (107). After the food was removed, you can see the two fractured halves, which were pushed even further apart as the horse chewed, forcing food between them.

Below left:
The two halves of the tooth after its extraction (from a standing horse).

Below right:
Sometimes part of the tooth is broken into bits: all separate pieces must be removed and carefully laid together to ensure that nothing is missing.

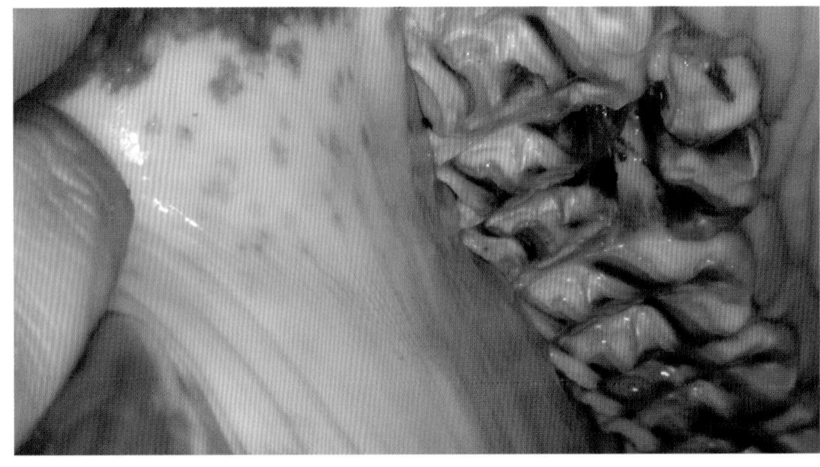

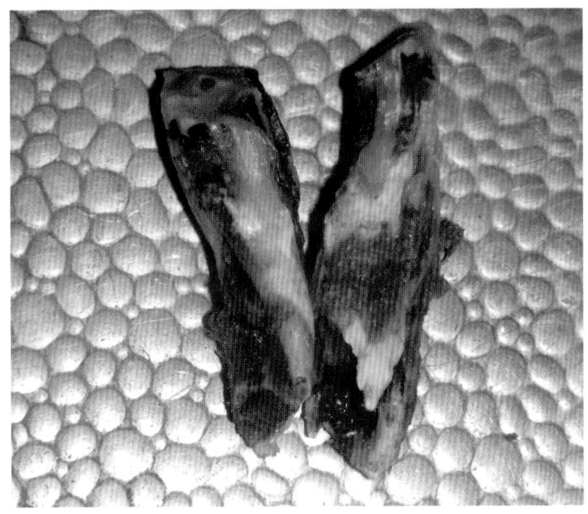

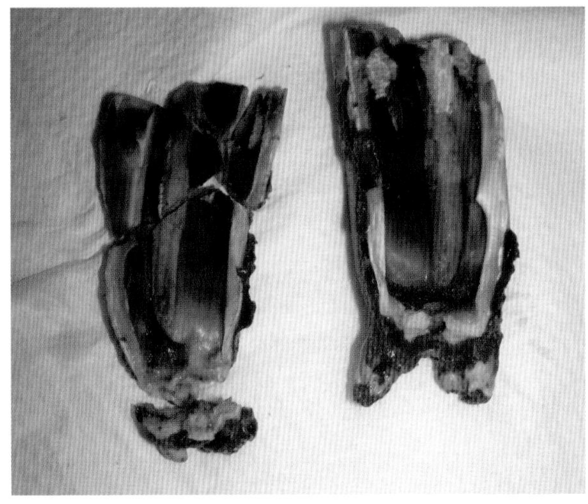

Both halves of the fractured tooth can usually be removed from the mouth while the horse is standing. If one of the halves is very fragmented, it is sometimes necessary to remove the remains under general anesthesia.

Sometimes little bits of the molar break off. This is usually of no consequence but if the top of the root canal becomes exposed, it could lead to the root canal becoming infected.

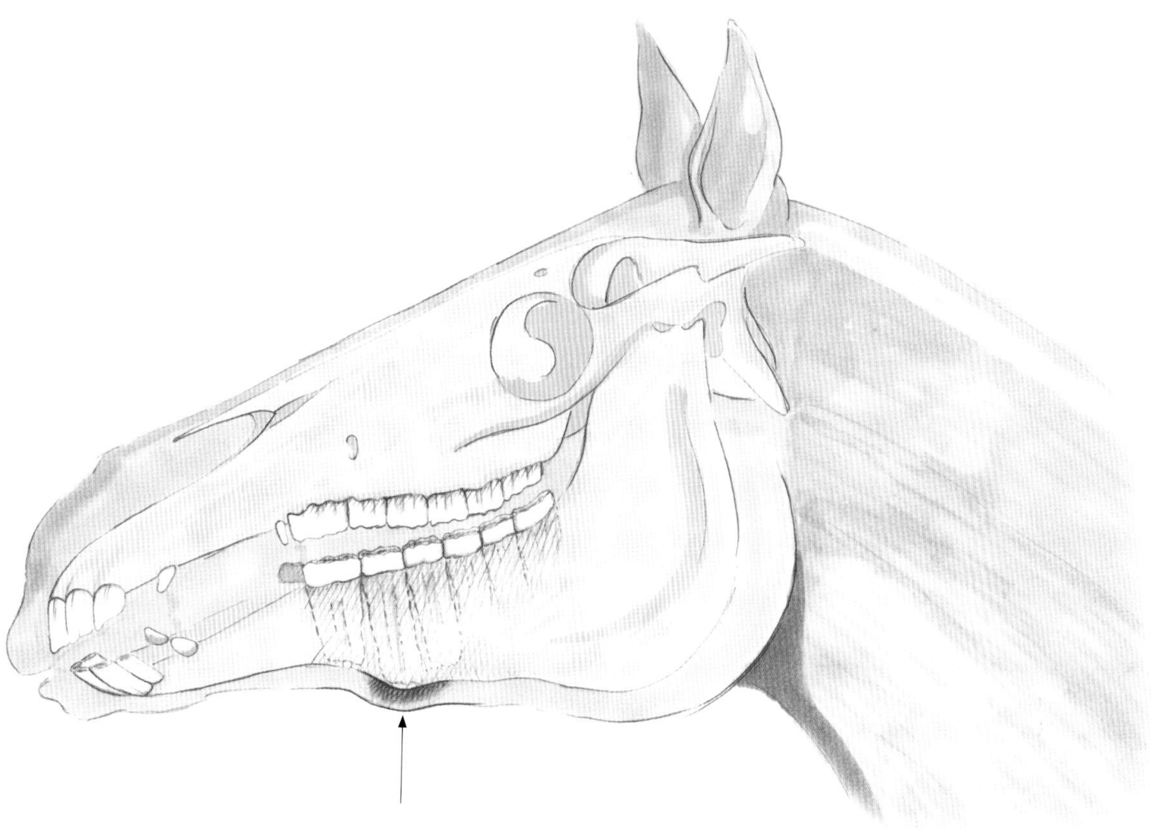

The swelling on the underside of the jaw in a young adult horse is called a mandibular bump.

Mandibular Bump

A mandibular bump is a thickening on the lower edge of the lower jaw—the mandible—that is caused by the roots of the permanent second or third molar. As the molar develops in the lower jaw and even before it erupts into the mouth, pressure from this tooth is created in the jaw bone from both the root end and the top end. The bone becomes thinner and gets pushed down from the pressure of the growing tooth on the lower side of the jaw bone. This bump sometimes appears at the age of 3-to-4-years old; it usually slowly disappears again in the following year as the tooth gets pushed up into the mouth.

The same process can be seen in the upper jaw. These bumps are seldom observed on the outside of the head due to the muscles present in this part of the head.

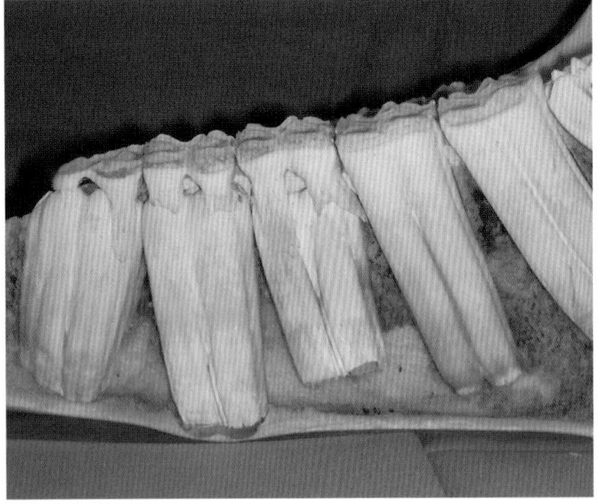

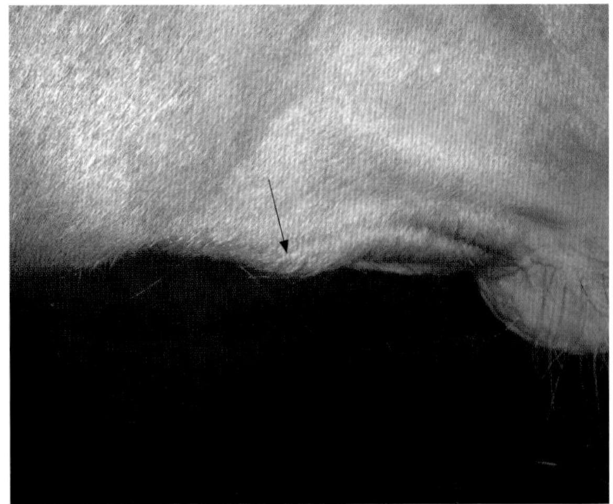

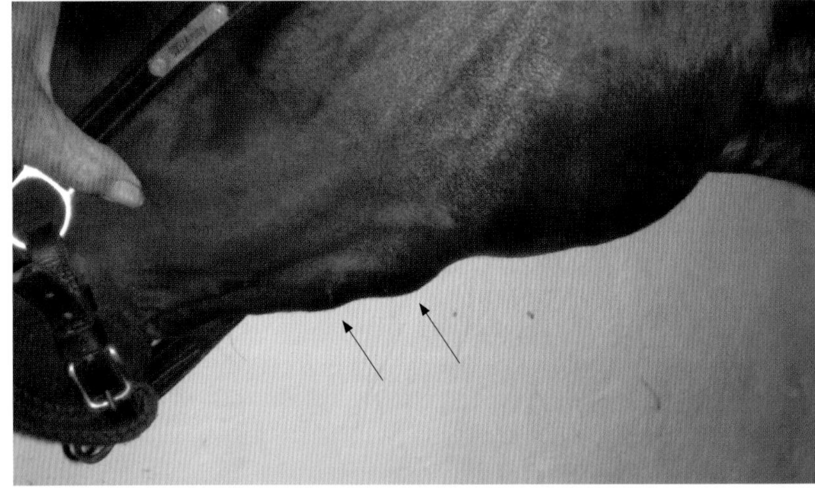

Top left:
A mandibular bump. The root of the permanent second molar presses on the jaw bone during the replacement process, and the jaw bone is forced downward. The bone has become much thinner at this spot.

Top right:
This swelling on the lower jaw of this three-year-old is a mandibular bump. The bulging of the bone is caused by the pressure from the root on the jaw bone during the replacement to permanent teeth; it will disappear within a year.

Below:
In this three-year-old, two mandibular bumps can be seen on the underside of the jaw. The roots of the second and third permanent teeth are responsible for the jaw bone bulging out.

Root Canal Infections

Sometimes a bacterial infection arises in the root of a tooth. This infection can reach the root in various ways: along the outside of a tooth by serious periodontitis; via the molar by the opening of the top of the root canal; and, infrequently, via the bloodstream from a trauma on the outside of the head such as a mandibular bump.

Depending on which tooth is involved, this can lead to sinusitis or the development of a tooth fistula.

Sinusitis

In the young adult horse, the roots of the last three to four upper molars lie against the base of the first and last maxillary sinuses—two cavities in the forehead. If a bacterial infection arises in the root of one of these teeth, then this can enter into the base of the sinus and can cause sinusitis—a bacterial infection of the sinus. This often shows as a suppurating and chronic one-sided runny nose. The causal tooth must be removed and the sinuses must be opened and cleaned. This usually takes place in a horse clinic under general anesthesia.

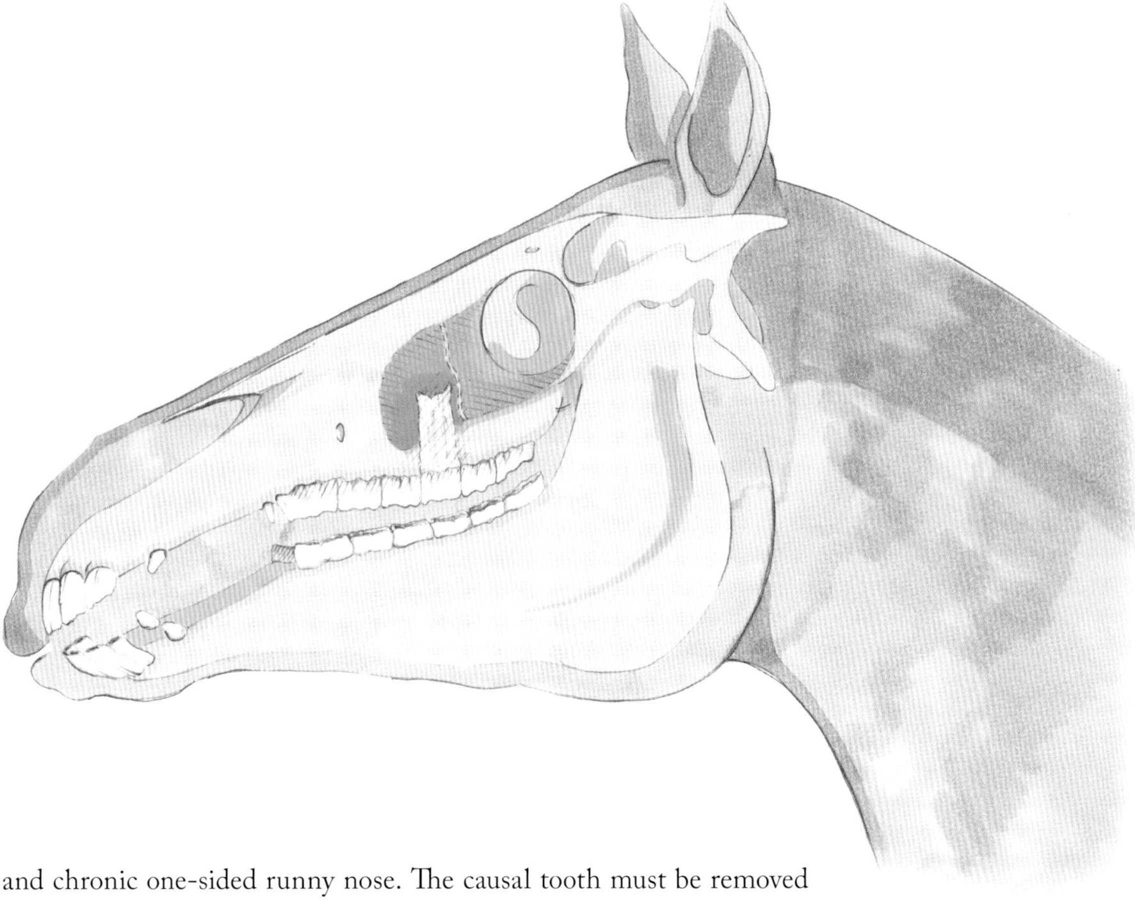

A dental root infection in one of the last four upper molars is often the cause of an infection in the neighboring sinuses in a young horse. You can usually observe a runny suppurating nostril on one side and sometimes, at the level of the sinuses, a swelling on the outside of the head.

Dental Fistula

If a root canal infection arises in the first two or three upper molars or in the lower molars, this infection often makes its way to the outside

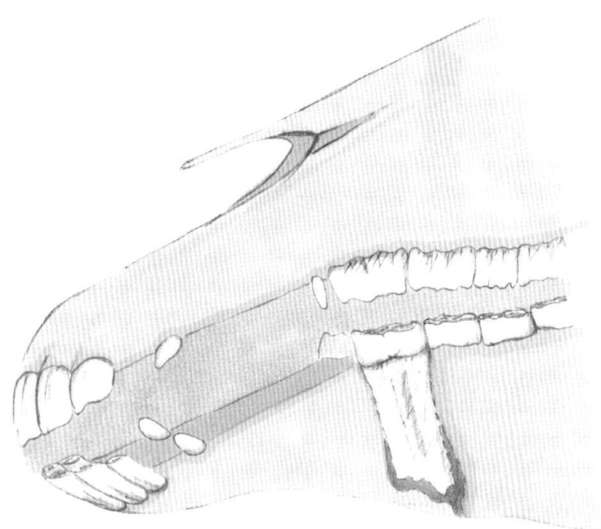

A dental fistula is an infection of the dental root that breaks through the jaw to the outside of the head.

through the bony socket of the tooth and the jaw bone. Then, an opening appears on the outside of the head often accompanied by emerging fluid or even pus. A fistula on the outside of the head at the level of the molars must be examined to find out if a tooth root is involved. This can best be done with X-rays. However, sometimes scintigraphy or a CT scan is needed to indicate the causal tooth. The table of the tooth affected often shows not the slightest sign of a defect. Establishing the tooth concerned merely from an examination of the set of teeth, is therefore usually not possible.

One can try to fight this infection at an early stage with long-term antibiotic treatment. This is often not successful and the teeth have to be removed anyway.

Top left:
Here you see a root infection of the first molar in the lower jaw (106) that has broken through the lower jaw in the form of an abscess. In order to solve this problem, the tooth usually has to be completely removed.

Above right:
A CT scan at the level of the fourth molar: on the right, you can see the roots of this molar (M) that reach up to the base of the sinus cavity (SC). On the left, the cavity has filled with pus (P) as a result of a dental root infection of the fourth upper molar. This is called suppurating sinusitis.

Below (both pictures):
Since he was three years old, this 12-year-old pony has shown suppurating dental fistulas of the third molars (107 and 207) on both sides of his head. Apparent lack of funds meant that he was not operated on, but the pony does not seem to have suffered.

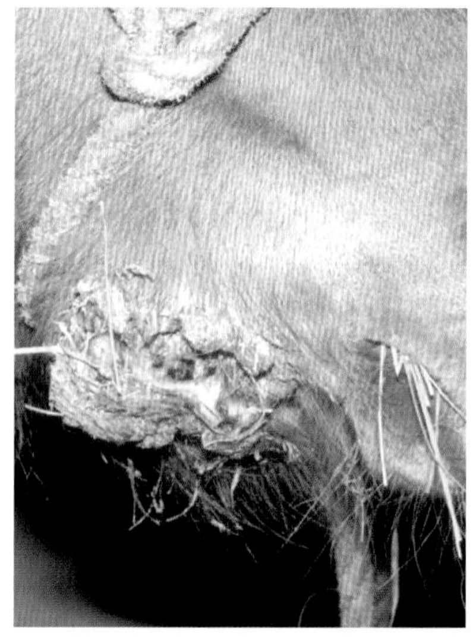

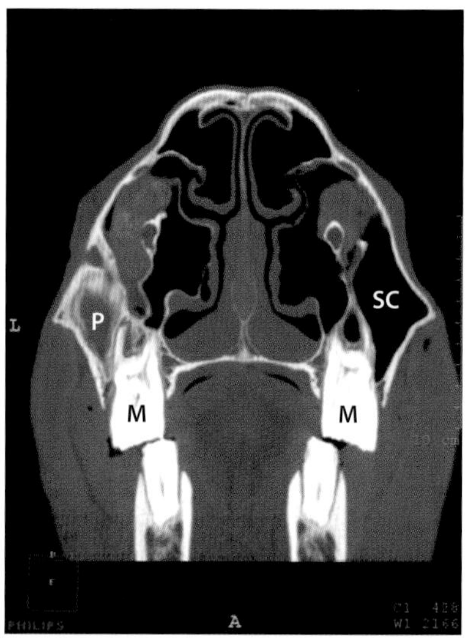

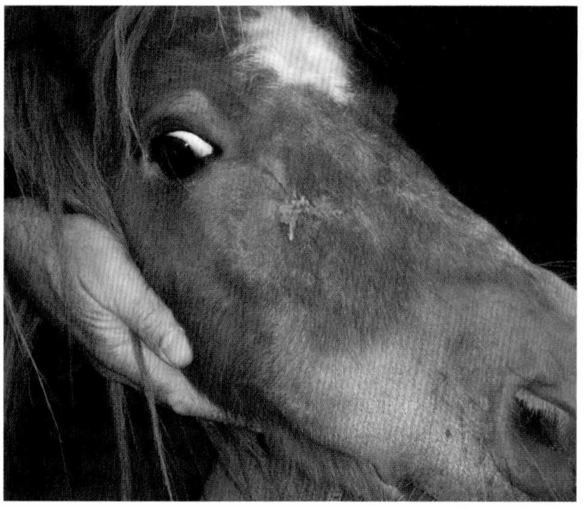

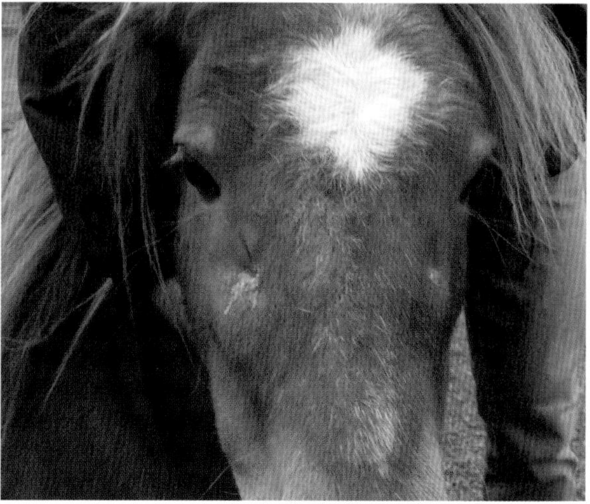

CHAPTER 12

Congenital Defects of the Set of Teeth

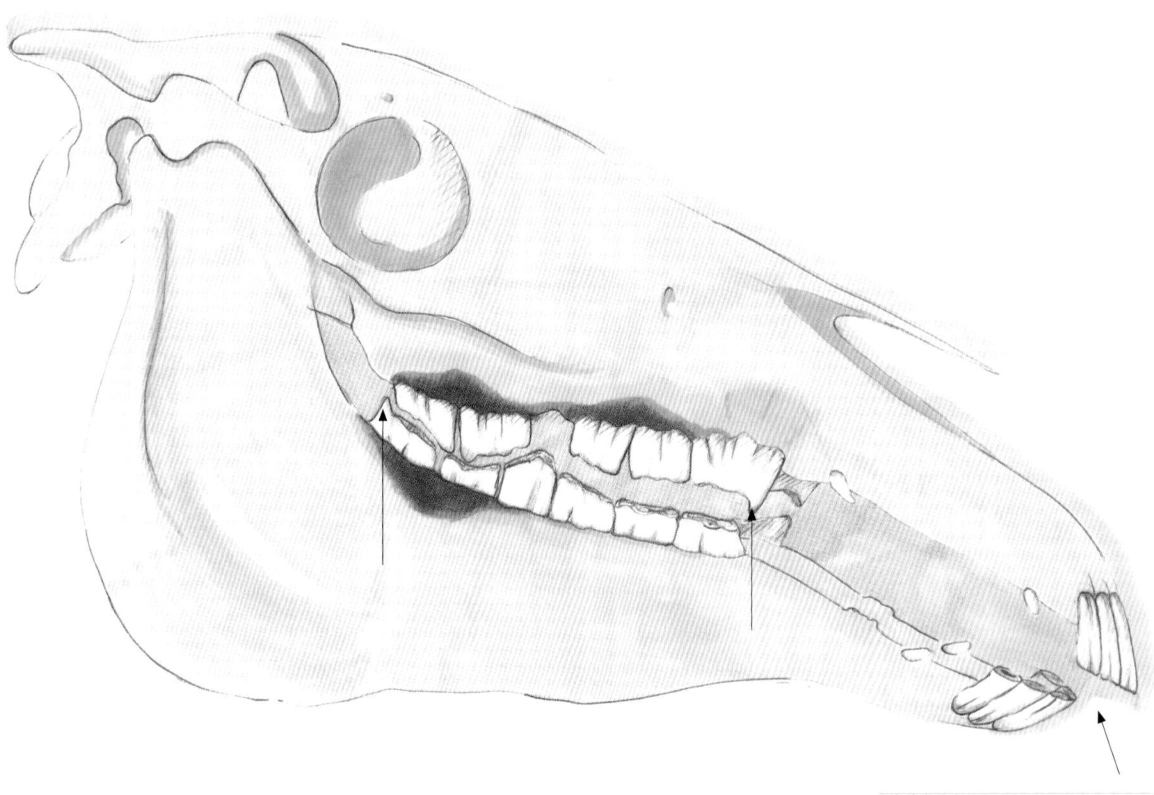

When the upper incisors jut out further than the lower incisors, it's called an "overbite." This often goes together with a front hook on the first upper molar and a back hook on the last lower molar.

Overbite

In an overbite the nipping edge of the incisors do not meet as they should: the incisors of the upper jaw jut further forward than those of the lower jaw. This can be just a couple of millimeters in front—where the back edge of the upper incisors still rest on the front of the lower incisors—or as much as three centimeters in cases where the upper incisors no longer meet the nipping edge of the lower incisors. Subsequently, the incisors become increasingly longer because their normal growth is no longer inhibited (worn down) from grinding action. The lower incisors then press into the palate behind the upper incisors. This is an inherited defect.

The lower incisors can become so long that the horse injures its hard palate behind the upper incisors. Very often, there is a related problem: usually the whole upper jaw is too far forward in relation to the lower jaw

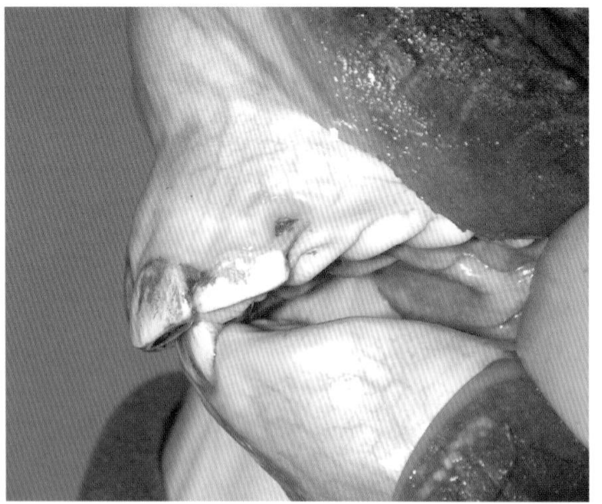

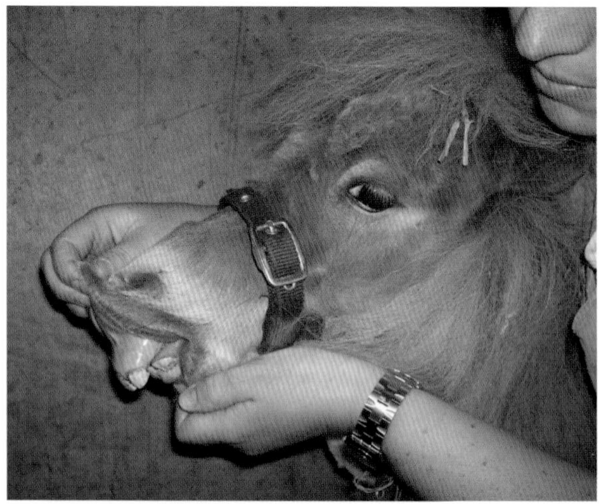

Top left:
A moderate overbite. The back edge of the upper incisors just touches the tables of the lower incisors.

Top right and middle:
This pony displays a serious overbite. The upper incisors jut several centimeters in front of the lower incisors. The incisors will get longer and longer as a result of lack of abrasion, and the lower incisors will then touch the hard palate.

Below:
The growth of the upper jaw can be controlled when there is a moderate overbite in foals; a brace that encircles the upper incisors and fixed on the first molar can hold back the forward growth of the upper jaw.

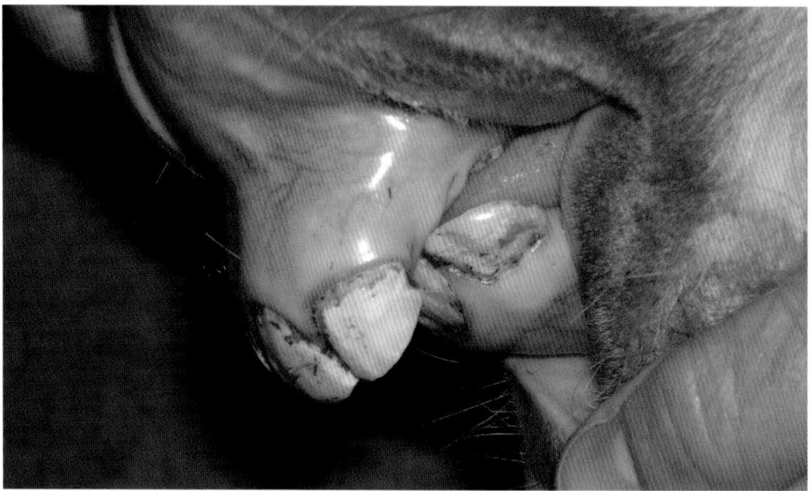

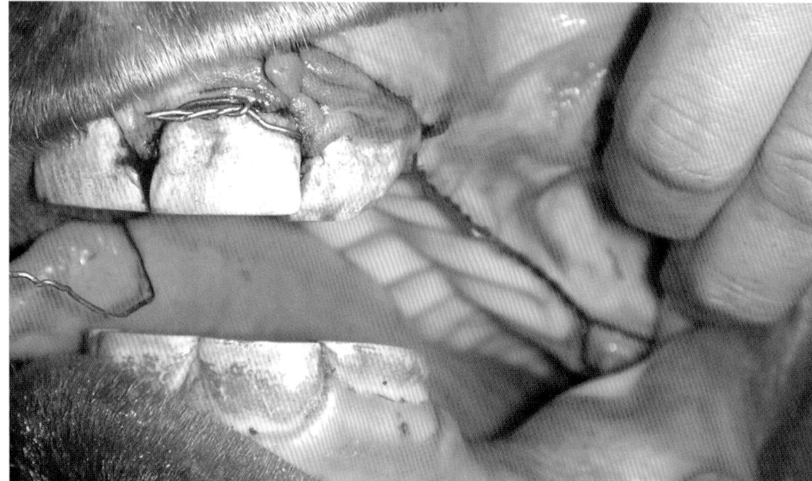

and a front hook develops on the first upper molars (106 and 206) and a back hook develops on the last lower molars (311 and 411). All these defects together are bound to produce a defective chewing cycle where the abrasion of the hooks becomes even less and, moreover, where other

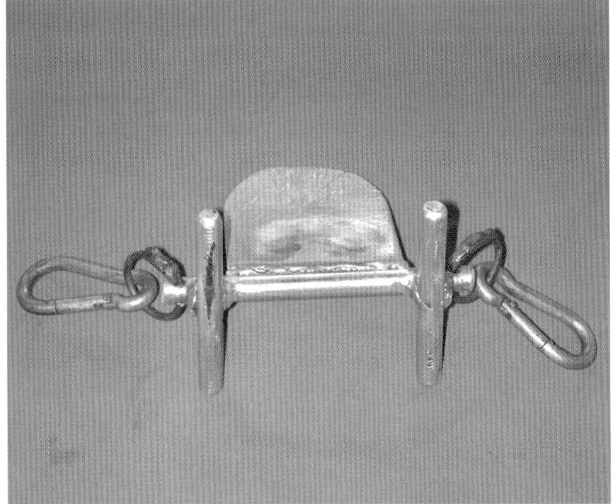

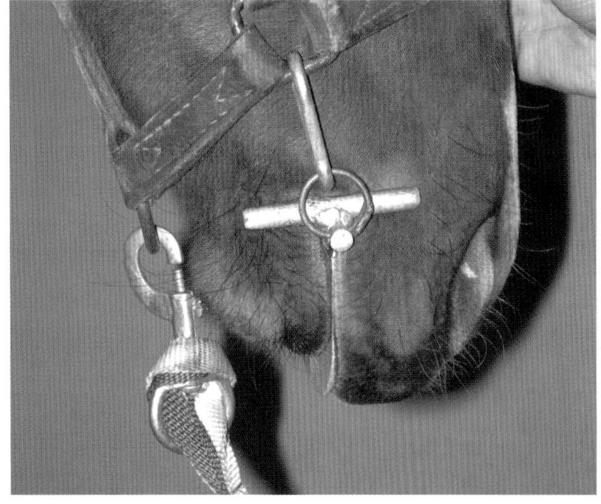

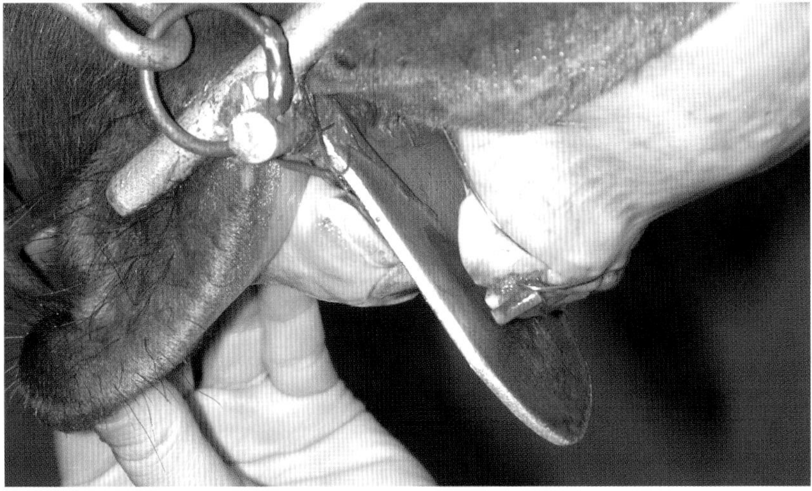

Top left :
As well as a brace, a "bite plate" has to be fitted in cases of serious overbite. This prevents the upper incisors from bending downward.

Top right:
A loose bite plate can be simply fixed to a halter. The bite plate must, however, be removed at feeding time.

Below:
A loose bite plate in the mouth of a six-month-old foal. This is combined with a brace that can be seen when the lips are opened.

defects can develop in the set of teeth. A yearly examination is absolutely necessary in this case. When a horse with an overbite is properly treated, this disorder will not pose any further problems either with his food intake or when being ridden.

If this defect is diagnosed at a young age, corrective treatment is a possibility. Due to the high cost involved, this is usually only carried out in genetically valuable foals. After a successful intervention, these animals are sometimes put through performance and young horse testing with the intent of acquiring breeding approval without the genetic defect being visible. Then an ethical problem arises because this intervention should really be mentioned in the stud book concerned; it is an inheritable defect and these animals should not be used for breeding.

If the upper incisors still touch the lower incisors, the incisor arc of the foal can have a brace of surgical metal wire fixed to the first molars from the age of three months. This will impede the forward growth of the upper jaw. As soon as good results are seen, the brace is removed. If the upper incisors really jut out in front of the lower ones, then the use of such a brace on its own would merely cause the upper jaw to bend in

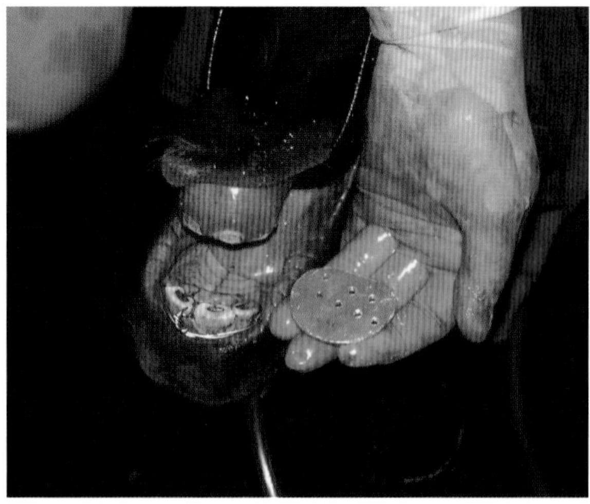

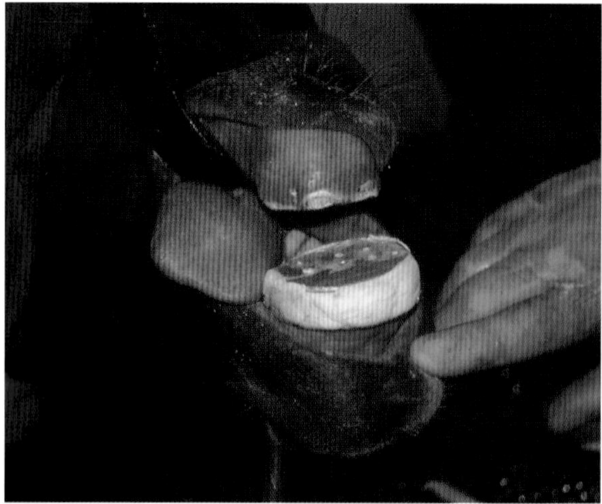

This is a picture of a foal with a serious overbite: an aluminium bite plate is fixed in the mouth with plastic.

front of the lower incisors. Such foals must also wear a loose bite plate or be fitted with an artificial bite plate against their hard palate. A loose bite plate is fixed to a bit and extends from the bit to the contact surface of the incisors. This has to be removed every time the horse is fed.

It is for this reason that sometimes a fixed bite plate is used. In this case, an aluminium plate is fixed with plastic to the brace onto the incisor tables of the upper teeth and the hard palate behind. The lower incisors can then supply the upward pressure needed.

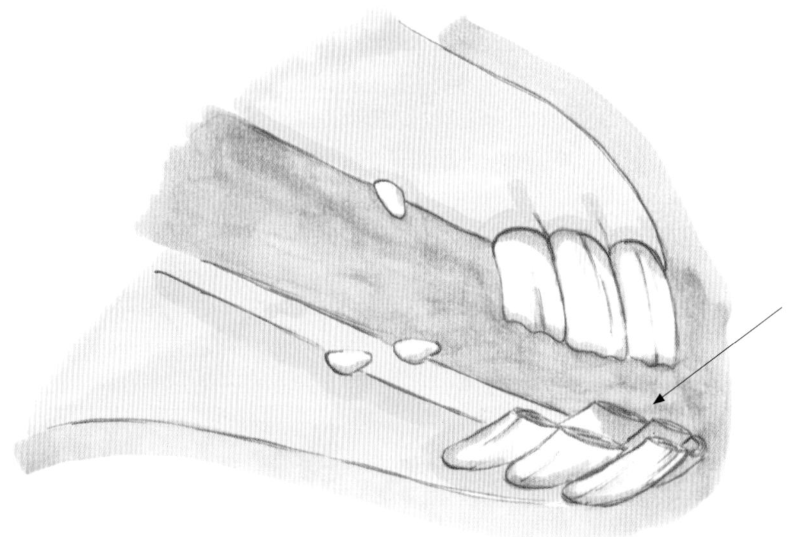

We call it an "underbite" when the lower incisors are further forward than the upper incisors.

Underbite

An underbite is when the lower incisors jut further forward than the upper incisors. This disorder is not seen as often as an overbite and is sometimes present in miniature horses. The same attendant dental defects can develop as the overbite but are in reverse. The first molars in

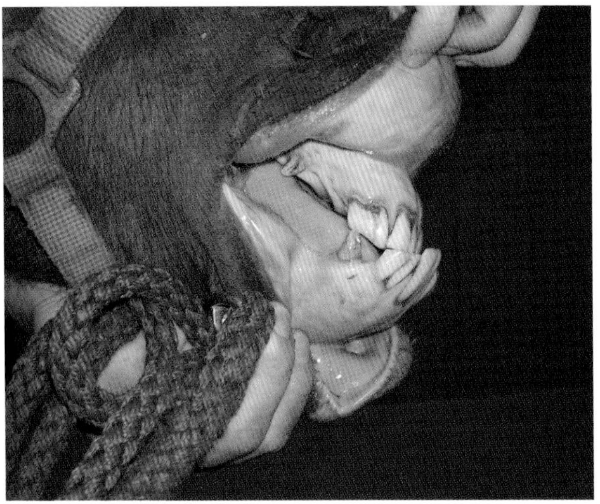

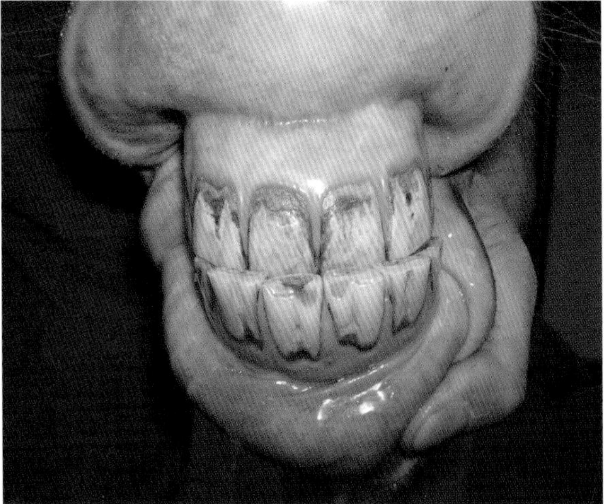

the lower jaw and the last molars in the upper jaw often develop hooks. In foals, an underbite is more difficult to treat than an overbite.

Top left:
A pony with a serious underbite. The tables of the upper and lower incisors do not meet: the lower incisors have become too long due to lack of abrasion.

Top right:
This is a picture of the same pony with the lower incisors cut back.

Too Many Teeth

Some horses have too many teeth. This is usually a seventh incisor or a seventh molar. This is caused by an abnormality in the development of the embryo: an extra tooth nucleus is produced that can later develop into a full tooth. As these teeth do not undergo any abrasion from the opposite arcade of teeth, which only has the normal complement of six teeth, they can grow beyond the normal table level and cause an upset chewing cycle.

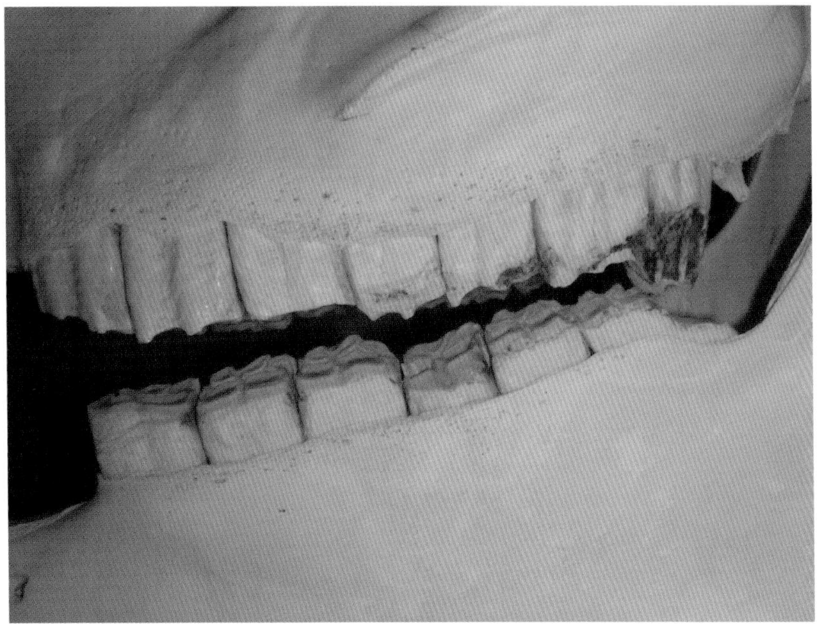

This horse had seven upper molars instead of the usual six. This has caused the back end of the last lower molar to become completely worn away. A step mouth is the result. This defect will certainly cause chewing problems in the long term.

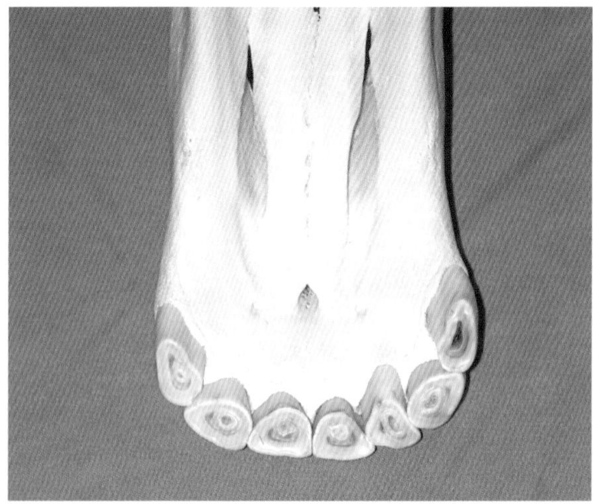

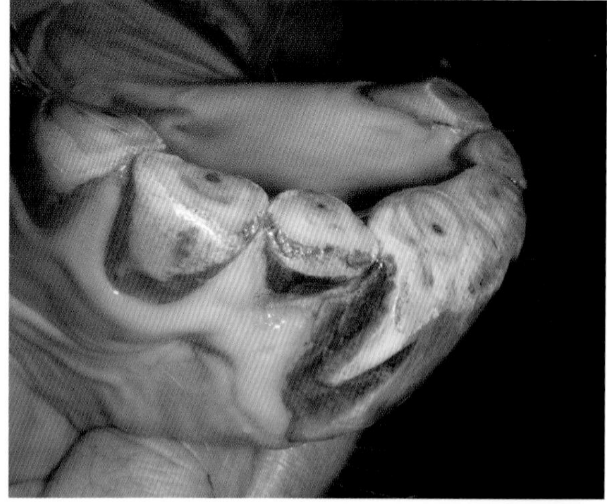

Top left:
The upper jaw of a skull that shows seven permanent incisors instead of the usual six.

Top right and middle:
This horse has six incisors in the lower jaw but the table of 301 appears to consist of two tables: the teeth have become united by dentine and are enveloped as one in a covering of enamel.

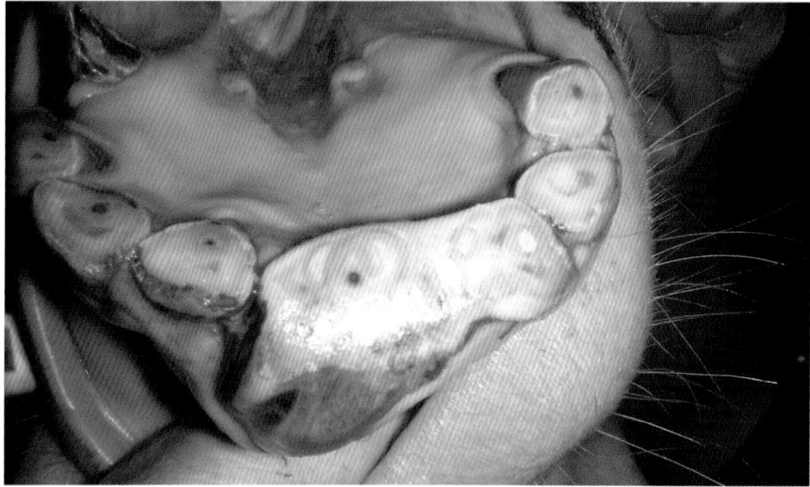

Too Few Teeth

Too few teeth as a congenital defect have rarely been recorded. What we do see often are older horses with this condition. Defects of the set of

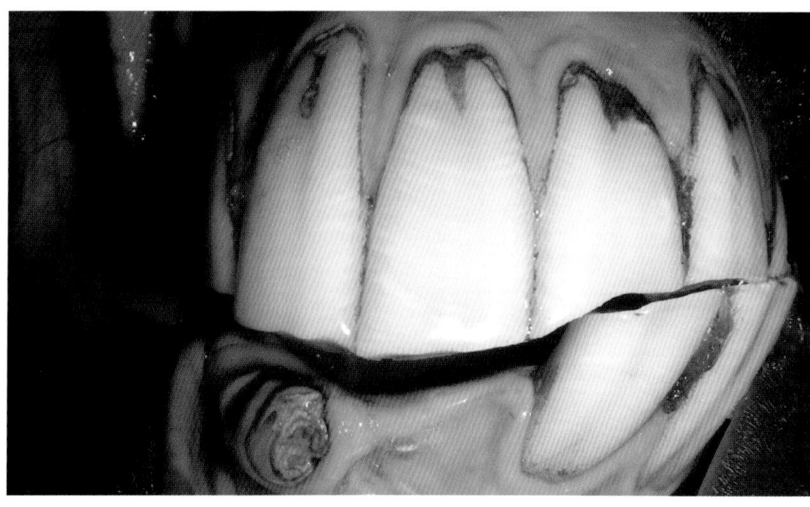

In the past, this 14-year-old horse lost three lower incisors of which only one still has the remains of the root (403). The lack of abrasion has resulted in the upper incisors growing down into the opening. The sideways-chewing movement of the jaw will certainly be hindered. The treatment consists of reducing the tables of the incisors concerned.

teeth as has been earlier described here can lead to molars—and occasionally, incisors—falling out or being extracted. Sometimes this can be as a result of external trauma with the breaking off of part of the socket with the accompanying incisor.

When there are missing teeth, the opposite teeth are no longer worn down and they grow taller and taller into the mouth. This will have consequences for sideways-chewing movement.

"Erratic" Teeth

An "erratic" or "ectopic" tooth is seldom seen. This is a tooth that, during the embryonic shifting of the teeth cells, remained behind and developed

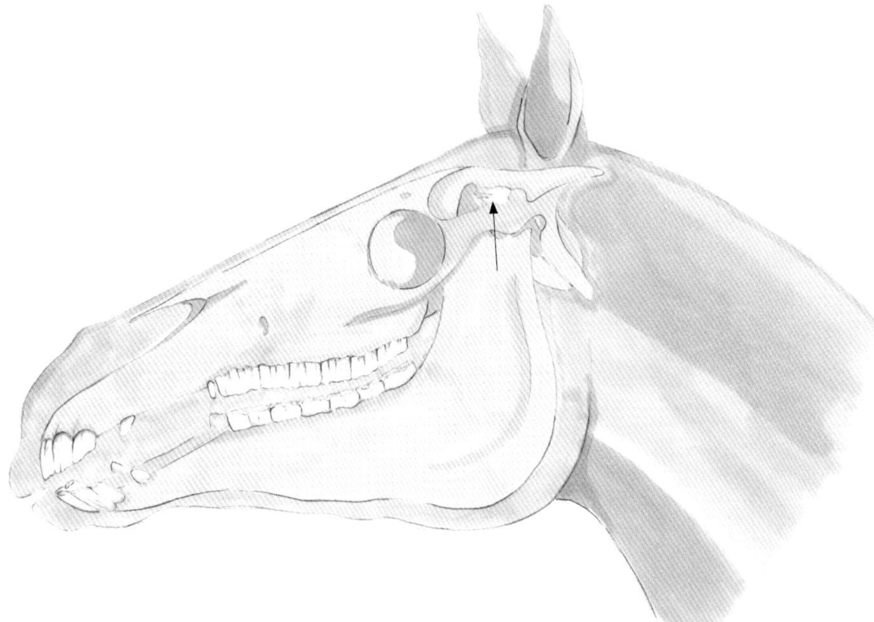

Top illustration:
A drawing of an "erratic" tooth that during the embryonic shifting of the teeth cells, remained behind and developed on the outside of the skull just in front of the base of the ear.

Below left:
A foal of three months with an erratic tooth that was diagnosed by X-ray. The secretion comes out through a fistulous opening on the front edge of the ear: it is produced by the mucous membrane that surrounds the erratic tooth.

Below right:
The extracted tooth was situated a couple of centimeters in front of the base of the ear against the skull.

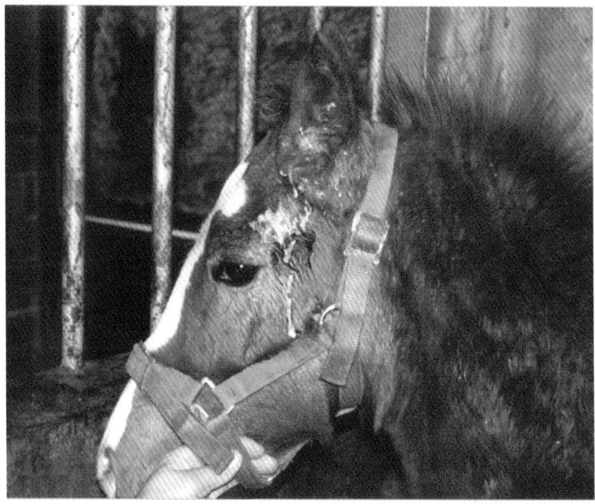

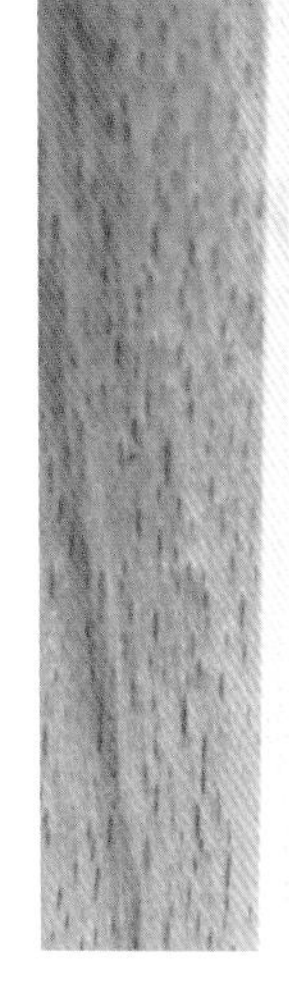

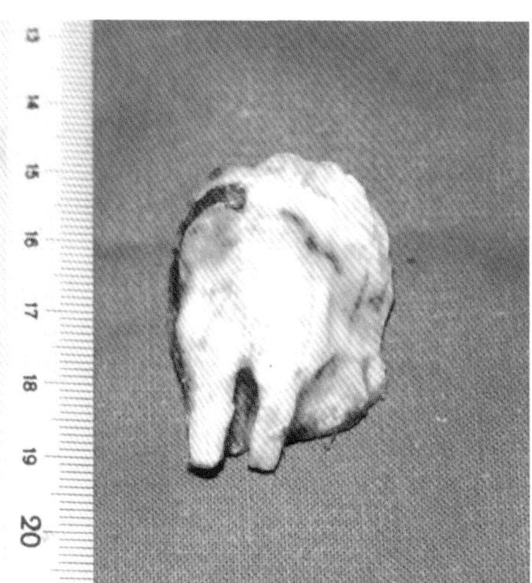

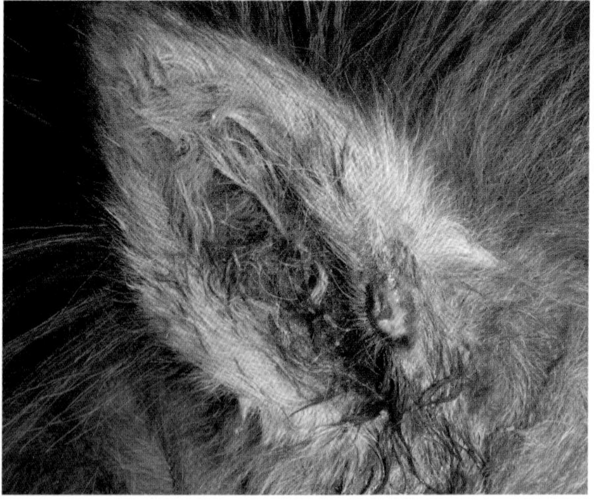

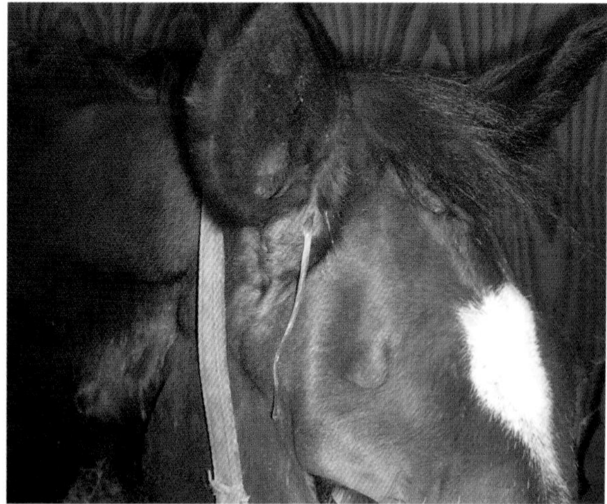

Top left:
A fistulous opening on the front edge of the ear nearly always indicates the presence of an erratic tooth.

Top right:
This horse has erratic teeth on both sides of its head. There is a regular secretion of slime from the fistulous opening in the ear.

against the outside of the skull at the base of the ear. This tooth usually has a small fistulous opening to the outside at the inner edge of the ear just above the forehead. A slimy secretion can exude from this opening and sometimes be excessive. When there is only a small discharge, regular cleaning is all that is needed. However, the only definitive solution is to remove the erratic tooth, which must be undertaken under general anesthetic in a clinic.

Asymmetrical Head

Below left and right:
A pony with an asymmetrical head. It is clear that the nose is bent to the left side of the head. Moreover, it has an underbite: the upper incisors are behind the lower incisors and are placed two centimeters to the left.

An asymmetrical head or bent nose has grown to one side so that the upper and lower incisors do not neatly fit together. This can vary from a minimal bend or a bend of several centimeters. In serious cases, it can also cause breathing difficulties due to partial blocking of the nostrils.

This defect is mostly seen among Arab horses and the smaller breeds. A

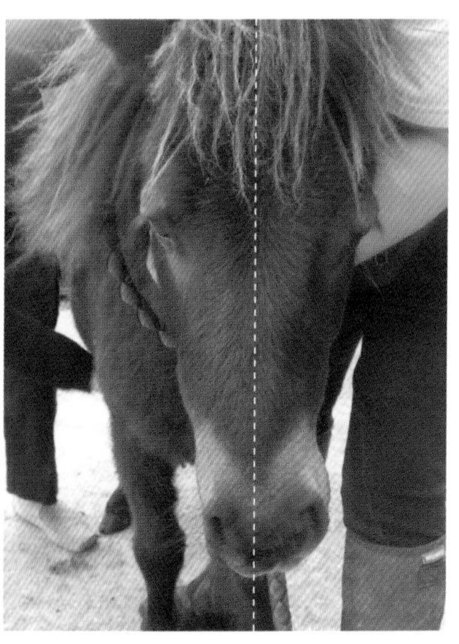

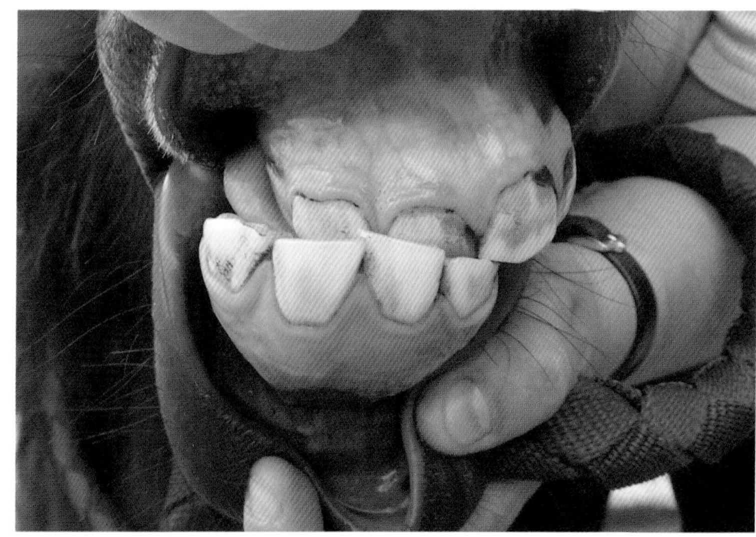

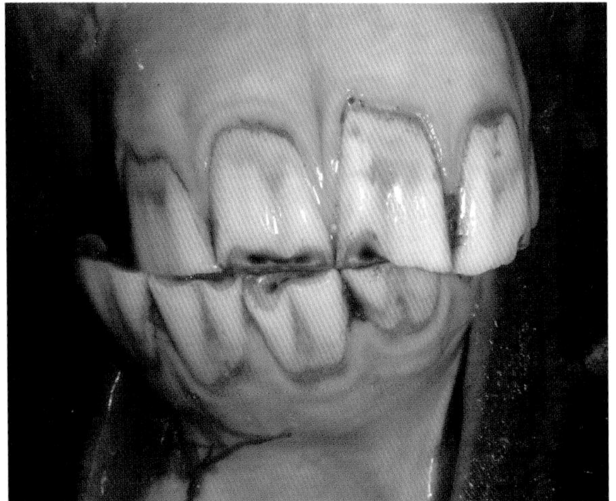

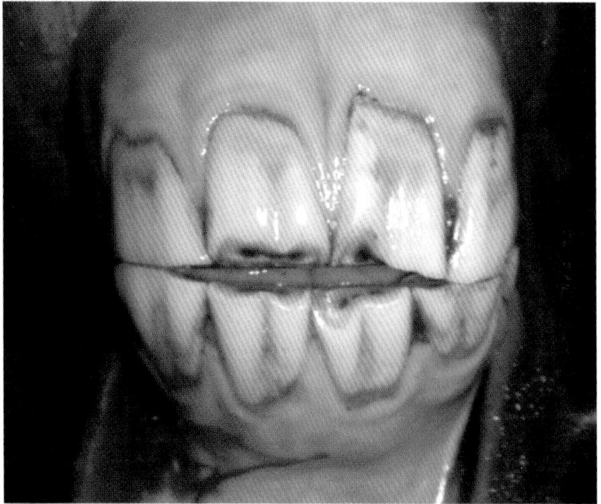

Top left:
A picture of an adult horse with an asymmetrical head. The corner upper incisors meet at the central lower incisors.

Top right:
If the incisors are "forced" into the correct position, the irregularity of the wearing down of the incisors is made clear.

poor position inside the womb could be responsible for the distortion.

If the defect is limited, these animals can be helped by regular dental care. As the incisors and the first molars do not fit properly together there will indeed be abnormal growth and abnormal abrasion.

In serious cases of an asymmetrical head with breathing problems, you can try to have the nose repositioned properly opposite the lower jaw with an operation. However, this is a complicated surgical intervention.

CHAPTER 13

The Dental Examination

The basis for every successful treatment is a clear and exact diagnosis. Therefore, it is essential to perform a thorough examination in order to be able to establish the correct dental treatment. Often, this procedure is still not respected.

A thorough dental examination must be carried out in a structured way. This can vary among dental technicians but the examination must be designed in such a way that all structures of the mouth are checked. A poor quality dental speculum and a feeble source of light make it impossible to conduct a good examination. A too rapid examination can mean that many defects in their early stages are overlooked. All too often a general examination consists of quickly looking into the horse's mouth by opening its lips and pushing the tongue between the molars. This only gives a superficial view of the incisors and the first molars and can hardly be called a thorough dental examination. A complete exam consists of feeling and looking at all hard and soft tissues within the mouth.

Defects in the mouth often remain undiscovered although they frequently exist. Indeed, many horses have never seen a dental technician and others have not had a proper dental examination. Actually, there is a big difference between the percentage of horses where a defect has been diagnosed and the percentage of defects that are found among slaughtered horses. The symptoms that a horse with dental defects shows are often not very specific, for example being a little resistant when being ridden and slight weight loss. It is because of this that sometimes help is called in only much later and when the symptoms are much more apparent, such as quidding. Unfortunately, things are often overlooked in an inadequate examination. When, for example, the source of light is poor, it is seldom possible to see a defect.

The aim of the dental examination is to discover possible defects at an early stage. These can then be corrected before irreparable damage is done to the set of teeth.

Security Measures

Before the commencement of the examination, it is important to ensure there is a good and safe working environment. This can be the horse's stall or box, the aisle between the stalls or an area designated for grooming. Make sure there are no objects lying around that could injure the horse. It is also advisable to have sufficient room above the horse's head. For various reasons it is not practical to examine the horse outside: when inserting the speculum and working on the teeth, the horse has a tendency to step backward. If this happens outside, there is no end to the distance it can go. Moreover, when you need extra light in the mouth, there is a totally different aspect to it outside than when working inside. For example, when you, yourself, have the sun in your eyes, your pupils will contract and less light falls on the retina. You can check this by looking into the beam of a pocket flashlight or torch outside in the sunshine and again in the dark.

The floor must not be too slippery (anesthetized horses are more likely to slip) and must be clean enough to be able to work hygienically. Then, with running water and electricity available, the examination can begin.

Dental Examination Equipment

I always begin by changing the horse's halter. Its own halter is usually prettier than mine but frequently has less room under the noseband. When the mouth is opened, such a noseband presses the cheek against the first molars. A thorough examination of these teeth is then virtually impossible, let alone giving treatment. It is better that the horse is not tied up but held by the lead rope instead. A horse that is tied up will—in a defensive reaction of the head—feel resistance: this may cause it to react even more strongly.

During a visual examination, the horse's head is best held at eye level. This can be done by resting the horse's head on the shoulder of the owner, but this is clumsy and dangerous. Should the horse make a deflecting movement, the horse's head or the speculum could cause serious injury

Left and right: The horse's head can be safely and easily held in a raised position with an adjustable dental stand. The lower jaw of the horse rests comfortably on the top of the stand and the mouth is then conveniently at eye level for the examination and any possible treatment.

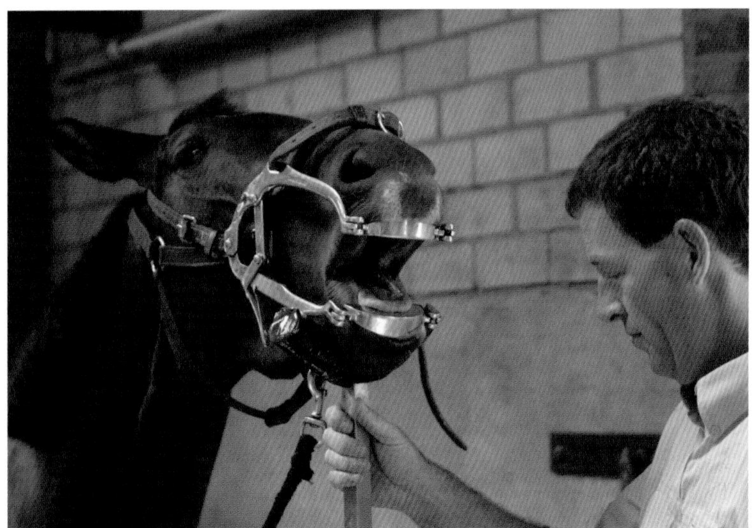

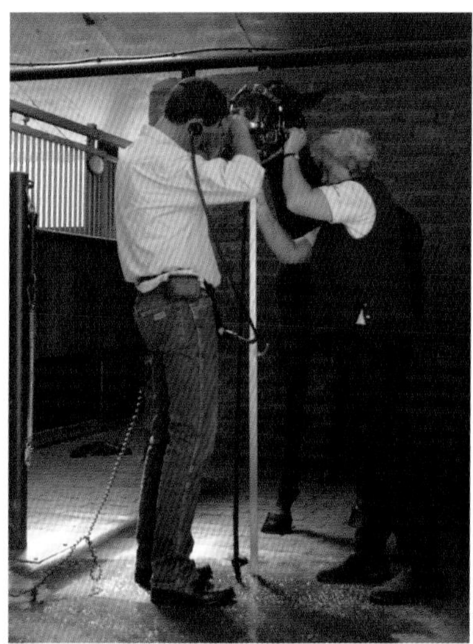

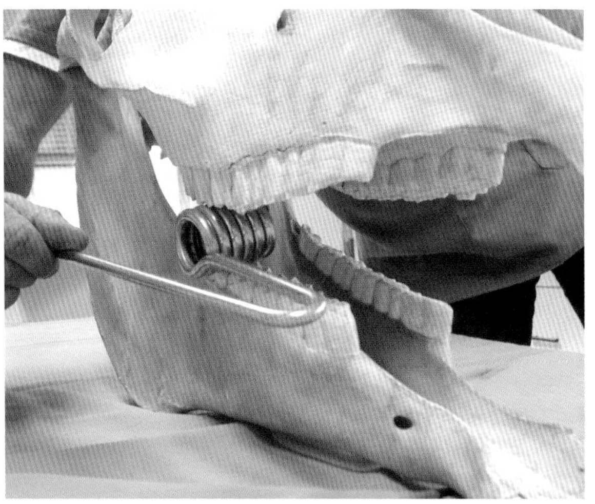

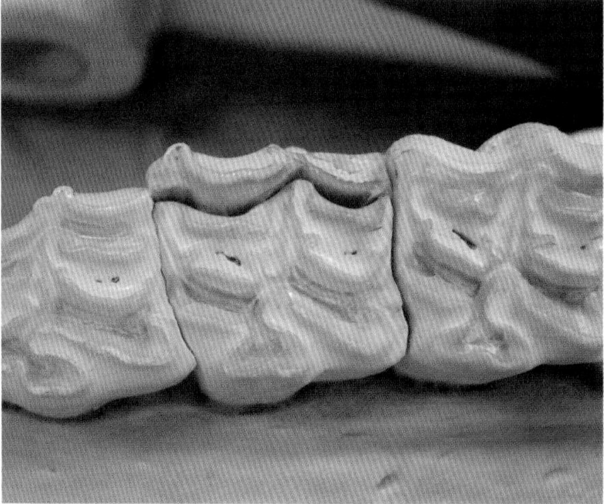

to the owner. Moreover, it is not pleasant to bear the weight of 45 to 50 lbs (20 to 25 km) on your shoulders for a half hour; and definitely not if there are four more horses also waiting for their turn.

Instead, we make use of a head support. There are two sorts: suspending head supports or dental stands. The suspending head support is used with a specially made halter. The noseband is strengthened with a metal brace round the nose with a ring attached in front above the nose. The horse's head is raised by putting a rope through the ring and by being held in place via a pulley over a beam. Sometimes the upper beam of the stable door is used. The metal brace in the noseband prevents the noseband from pressing against the cheeks. The rope is belayed with a quick release knot so that with one pull, it can be released in the case of a calamity. The other head support—the dental stand—comes in all types. Basically, it is a pole with adjustable height and a V-shaped fixture at the top on which the lower jaw of the horse rests.

Left:
Use of a one-sided type of speculum is actually out of date. The horses continually chew on it, the view inside the mouth is extremely limited and it is dangerous for both the dental technician and the horse itself.

Right:
When using this type of speculum the full pressure of biting falls on the table of one single molar; the danger of fracturing the tooth is always present.

A good dental speculum is an essential piece of equipment for an examination. There are two types: the one-sided type and the full-mouth speculum. In the one-sided type, a wedge or a cylinder is brought between the upper and lower molars and held or tied in position by a brace. This wedge or cylinder can be made of metal or can be covered in rubber. This type of speculum is easy to insert but has a number of disadvantages. The horse, in a reflex action, begins to chew on the wedge. This makes a manual examination in the rear of the mouth cavity nearly impossible to carry out due to the risk of getting one's fingertips crushed. When the metal cylinder is inserted, the full biting strength comes to rest on the table of one molar: in this way, sometimes the outer edge of the molar can fracture. If the wedge slips out when the horse is chewing, the gums and the hard palate can be injured. Above all, the pressure on the hard palate of your horse is very painful. The tongue is pushed to the other side by the wedge, which blocks the view of the arcade of teeth on that side. It's clear that this sort of speculum is out of date and dangerous for your horse.

What is much more pleasant is the full-mouth dental speculum. The mouth is held open by metal plates on the tables of the upper and lower incisors. The pressure is thus dispersed over all 12 incisors. Horses that are familiar with a bit rarely display difficulties with the insertion of this type of speculum. Once this speculum is correctly inserted, the horse stands quietly without it being possible for it to make a chewing movement. The advantage of this speculum is ease of access to the whole mouth for both seeing and feeling. In the case of any treatment, the molars can also be quickly reached.

If an extensive treatment is called for, we close the speculum for a while every 20 minutes. This is done to prevent strain on the jaw muscle that could lead to the horse have difficulties eating for a couple of days

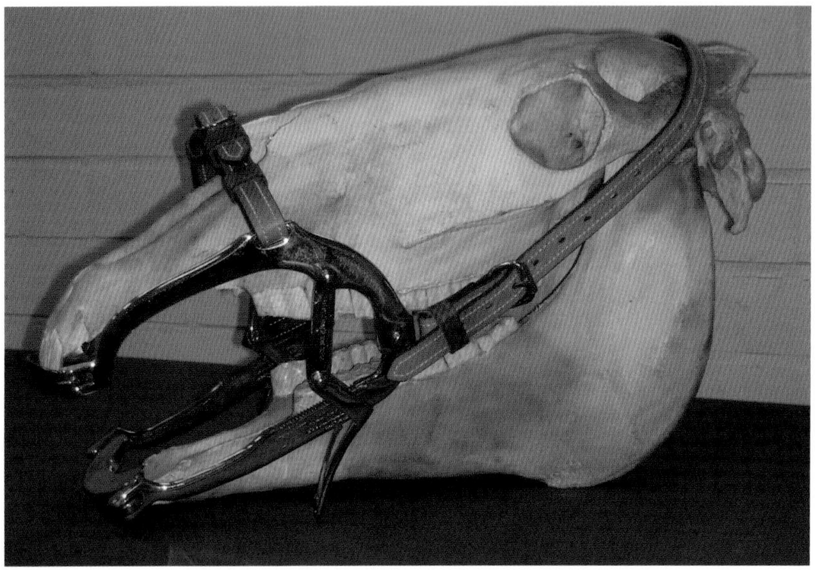

The pressure of biting is spread equally over all the incisors in the full-mouth dental speculum. This speculum is easy to insert, comfortable for the horse and allows maximum access into the mouth for both the examination and the treatment.

which, of course, you don't want to happen. If the horse becomes restless or continually shakes its head, a light anesthetic may be necessary for a thorough dental examination.

In order to see inside the mouth properly, a good source of light is needed. By that I mean more than just turning the mouth opening toward the sun. A small powerful pocket flashlight or torch gives good light but it is often in the way of a proper view. A forehead lamp offers totally free hands and shines the light where one is looking. To this end, there are even very powerful halogen lights with enormous illuminating power that have been developed. If you need to see something in the mouth there can never be too much light. There are also specially developed LED lamps that can be fixed on the speculum at the hard palate. These provide a constant source of light in the mouth independent from any movement made by the examiner. With a good light source and a dental mirror, a thorough investigation of the tables of the molars and the surrounding soft tissue is possible. In this way, caries, diastemas, periodontitis and other dental defects can be caught

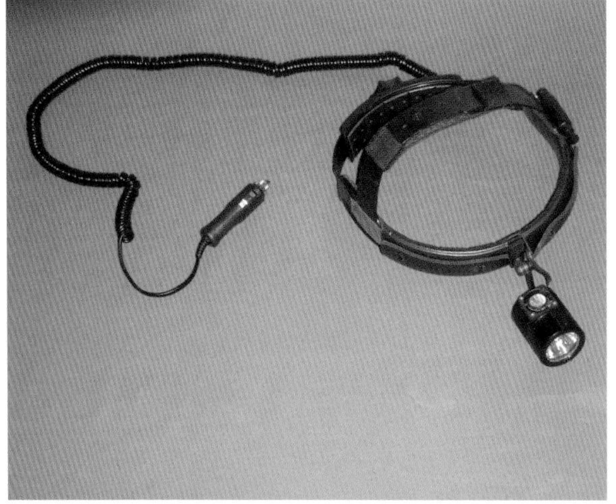

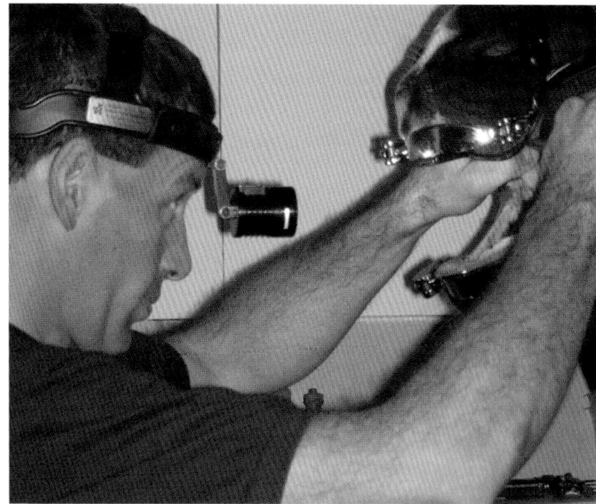

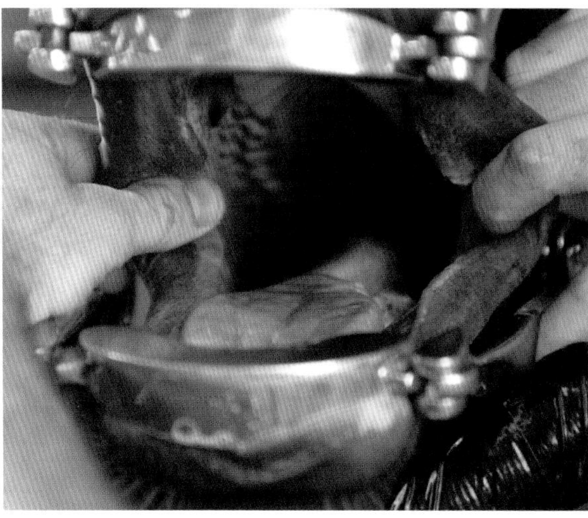

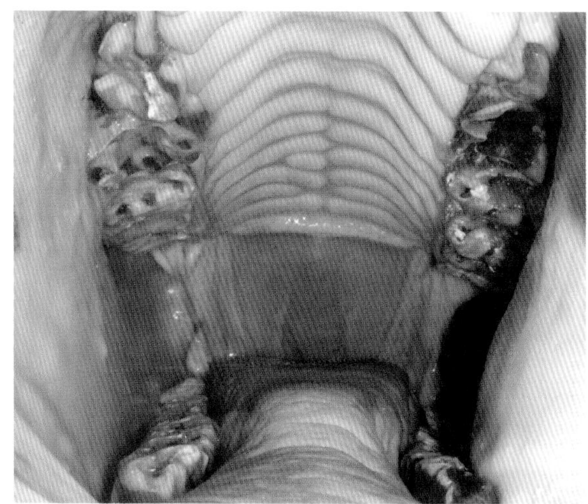

at an early stage. Long tooth picks are useful for the examination of diastemas or periodontitis.

Top left and right:
A good light source is an essential piece of equipment for a thorough examination of the mouth. This is a portable lamp with a powerful halogen bulb that has been developed for equine dental examinations.

Below left:
Without a light source, visual examination of the mouth is impossible: the technician is then looking into a dark cavity unable to distinguish separate molars.

Below right:
With a suitable portable lamp the inside of the mouth is fully illuminated.

Previous History

The discussion that the dental technician has with you while he or she prepares the equipment can provide him or her with a lot of insight. A horse that becomes fatter and fatter in the summer but loses weight in the winter is nearly certain to have a defect of the molars. When horses are nervous, a more careful approach is required. When broodmares are being examined, questions will be asked about any possible pregnancy. If anesthesia is necessary with broodmares then the dental treatment will be postponed during the last three months of the gestation period. Questions will be asked as to what type of discipline the horse is used for and what the competition schedule is. It is not wise to hastily have dental treatment a week before an important competition nor, for example, to have wolf teeth removed. The use of some medicines also test positive

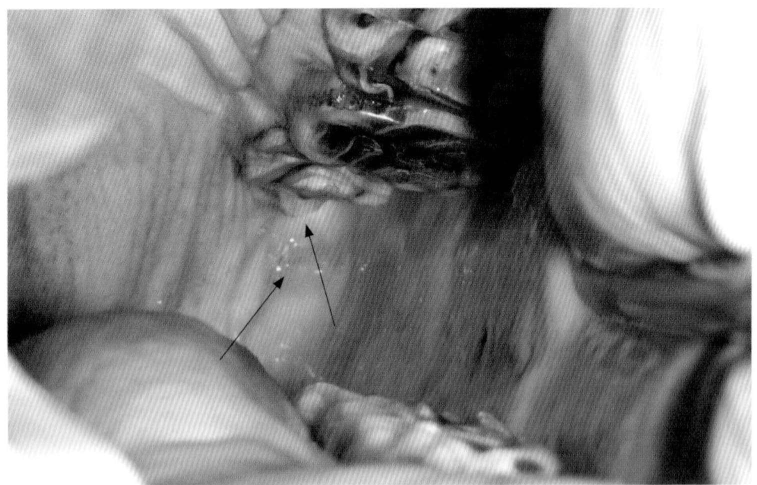

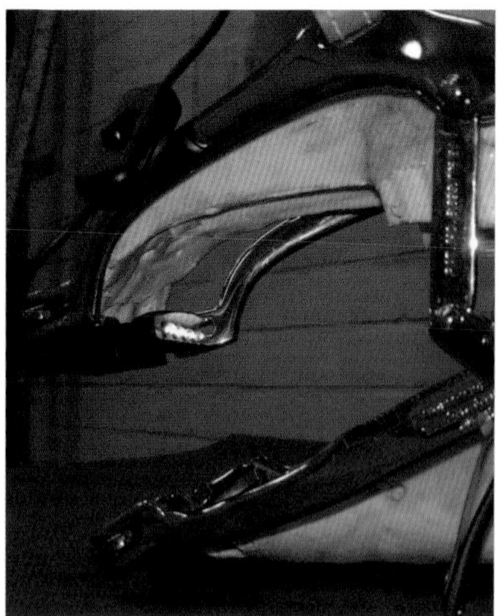

Left:
With a good light source the small rear hook on the last upper molar (211) and the dark patch of irritated soft tissue behind it are clearly visible. The removal of the hook on this dressage horse quickly solved its problems with leaning on the bit.

Right:
A light source, moreover, can be fixed behind the upper incisors: this makes examination of the inside of the mouth extremely easy.

in the doping controls of competition horses. It is better then that all this takes place in a quiet period on the competition calendar. Are there problems with riding on the bit? Or does the horse resist the bit? Is the mouth foam sometimes pink?

If your horse has already previously been examined or treated, then checking the former dental record will indicate what kind of problems there could possibly be. Horses that have previously had correction for a dental defect apparently have up to six times the likelihood of a new defect than the average horse.

What is the vaccination status of your horse? For example, removal of wolf teeth requires he is vaccinated against tetanus. If he has not been, then an anti-tetanus serum can be administered on the spot by a veterinarian.

Observation of the Horse

Observing the horse in the stable before commencing treatment is particularly useful when the complaints concern feeding or if the horse is too thin. The types of concentrated feed and roughage are considered: questions should be asked about the composition and the amounts of the ration. Sometimes, for example, a horse will not eat because it has a high temperature. In such cases, you would first have your horse examined and treated by a veterinarian. Some horses begin to eat greedily but then suddenly make a face and let the feed fall from their mouth. Some restless horses hang their heads over the stable door or look out of the window between every couple of mouthfuls; this can also result in spilled rations. However, this is seldom an indication of dental problems—most horses spill feed but when they have their head down in the feed bucket or manger, it is not noticed. If there are wads of dropped food in front of the stall or box door or on its floor–as explained earlier, an act called "quidding"—then the horse definitely has a dental problem.

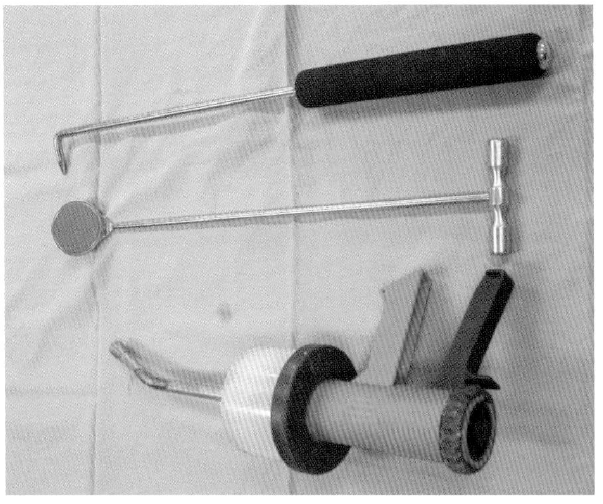

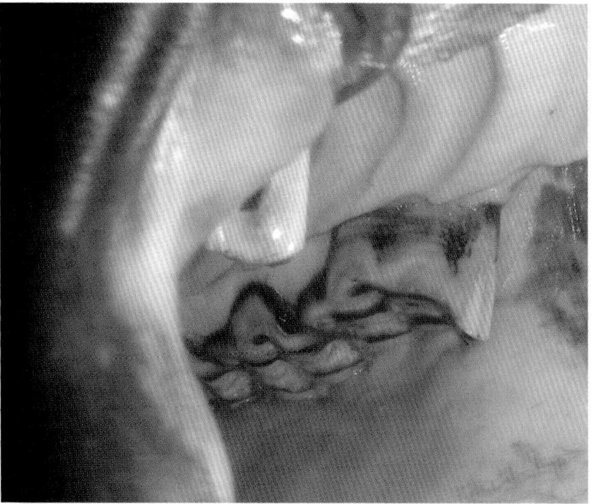

What does the horse's manure or dung look like? Sometimes it contains undigested grain or rather too long fibers that indicate an inadequate chewing cycle. Dental problems can also cause diarrhea or manure that is too dry, which leads to constipation.

By looking at the stall door or the edge of the feed bucket, you can sometimes observe whether the horse has stable vices. Horses that crib and/or windsuck usually take hold of the same object in the stable with their teeth. The metal or wood here is often then bright and shiny and wet. With such horses, you expect to see abnormal abrasion of the teeth.

Top left:
Equipment needed for an examination of the mouth: The large hand spray is used for rinsing food remains from the mouth. The dental mirror is used for making a thorough inspection of the molar tables. The toothpick loosens any remaining forage.

Top right:
A front hook on the first upper molar. This hook was easy to remove but, with this horse, it will reappear in the future. If records have shown that a horse had previously had a hook removed then the dental technician can pay extra attention at the following examination.

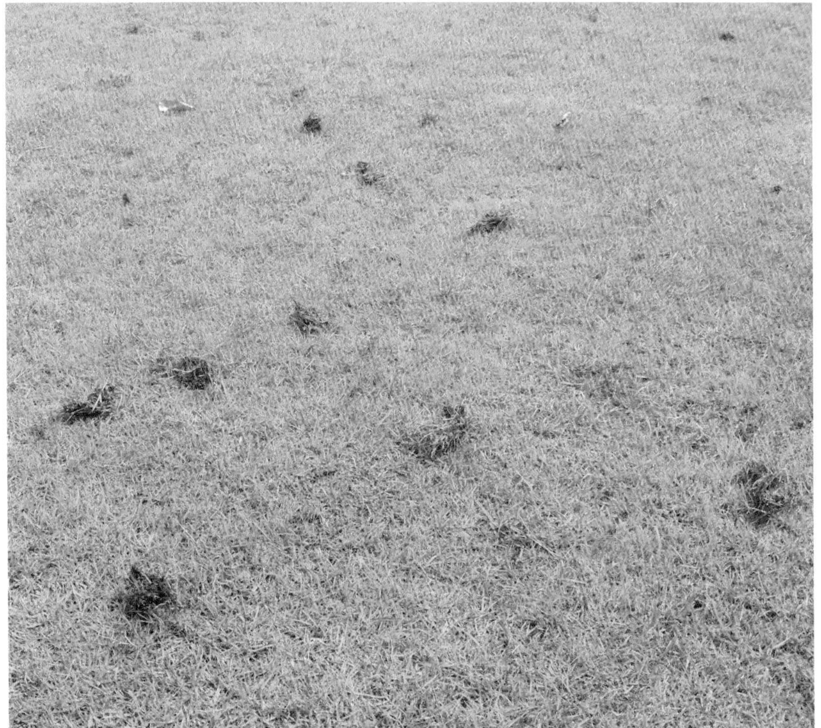

This pasture of a miniature pony is scattered with wads of dropped forage. Quidding always indicates serious problems in the mouth.

External Evaluation of the Head

During the external examination of the head the principle concern is the symmetry between the left and right sides. Asymmetry in the bony structure of the lower jaw can indicate an old healed fracture. Such a fracture can have disturbed the arrangement of the teeth. The chewing muscles should be well developed. Problems in the jaw joint can sometimes cause pain if there is pressure on the jaw joint. However, problems in the jaw joint seldom arise. Any swelling is examined and evaluated in relation to the set of teeth. The mandibular bumps on the underside of the lower jaw are a normal symptom in a four-year-old horse. Very, very occasionally, we see a horse with an asymmetrical skull where the nose is bent to one side. This is sometimes reflected in the position of the incisors.

Some horses have a clear swelling under the skin on the outside of an arcade of teeth. This is caused by the hoarding of food between the

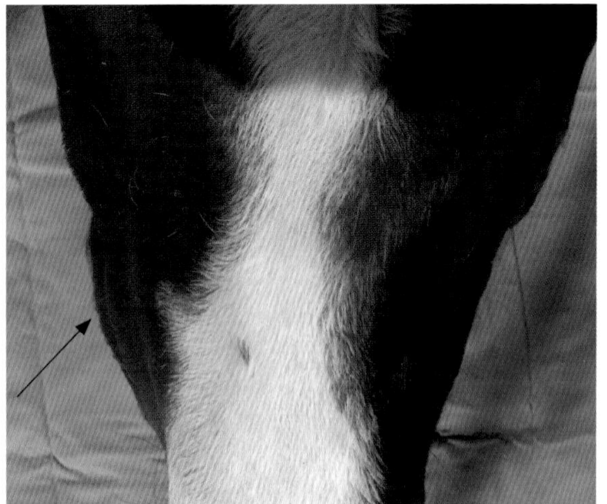

Left:
This horse shows a bulge in its right cheek caused by the squirreling of food. This always indicates a serious dental defect.

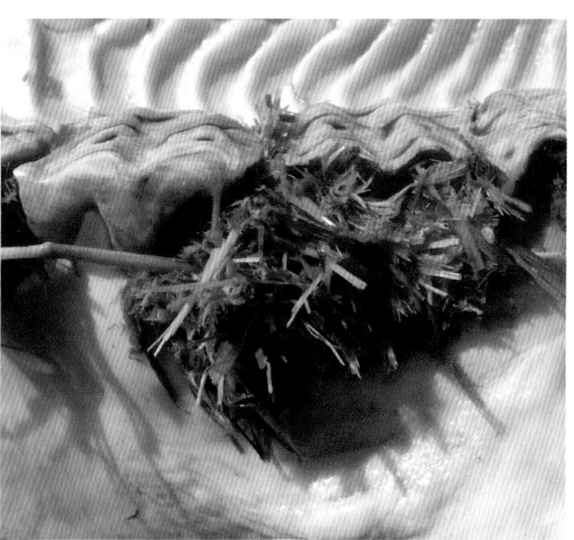

Right:
This particular bulge was caused by food that was stuck between several diastemas.

cheek and the outside of the molars and is called "squirreling": it often indicates a serious dental defect.

If there are signs of infection present such as a runny fistula (an opening on the outside of the jaws exuding pus) or a runny nose it is better to have this looked at by a veterinarian or the vet/dental technician first in order to establish its cause. A runny fistula on the lower jaw can be caused by either an erupted root infection of a lower molar or by a fracture in the lower jaw. In the latter, it is advisable to have an examination by a veterinarian before the speculum is inserted and opened; this can otherwise lead to a hair fracture becoming a full fracture of the jaw bone with catastrophic consequences.

A discharge of pus from the nose with a high temperature can indicate an infection of the upper respiratory tract; thus the dental examination and treatment can better be postponed until the horse has recuperated.

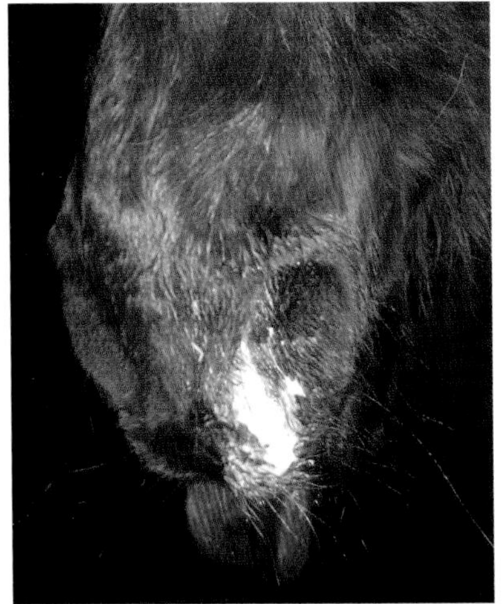

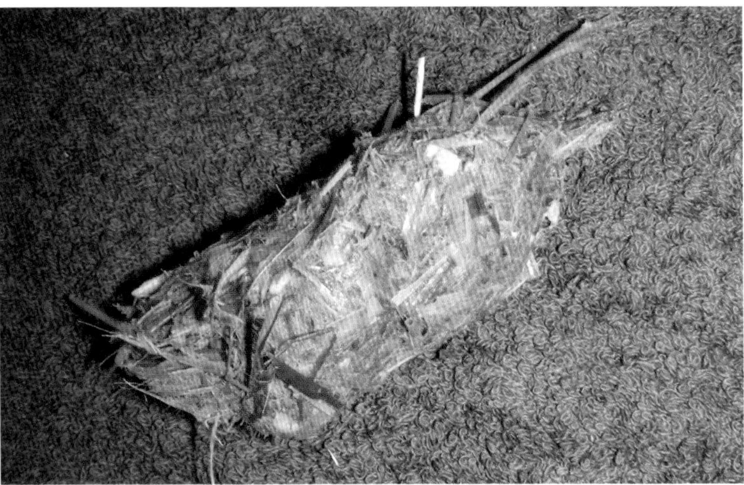

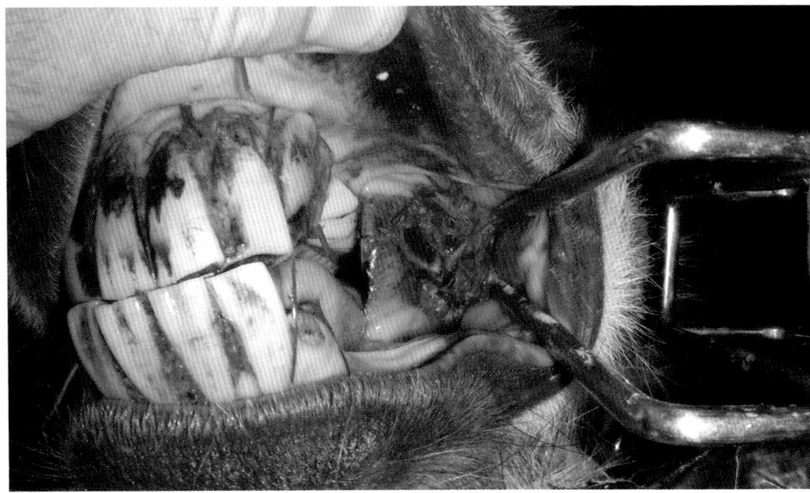

Top left:
A pony displaying a runny nose in the left nostril. This can indicate an infection in the upper respiratory tract or, less commonly, sinusitis as a result of a molar disorder. This 28-year-old pony turned out to have sinusitis. It had been caused by several diastemas between the last upper molars; the food between the teeth had been pushed up into the sinus cavity during chewing.

Top right and below:
When the cheek of this miniature donkey was pulled open, there was clear squirreling of food on the outer side of the first molars. When the mouth was opened for the examination, this wad of food of at least 8 cm fell out of the mouth. Here, squirreling was because of a loose second upper molar (107) that had been pushed into the cheek. The tables of the incisors are also very irregular.

A runny nose can also indicate a suppurating sinus as a result of a bacterial root infection of one of the four upper molars. In this case, a very thorough dental examination is needed in order to identify the molar causing the trouble. This is definitely an aspect where veterinary dental technicians have an enormous advantage over lay dental technicians. Veterinary dental technicians are far better qualified to judge the other symptoms as well as the dental defects and can see the overall picture. Thus the difference between a horse that cannot chew anymore and a horse that cannot swallow anymore is easier for a veterinarian to identify. Indeed, these two defects demand completely separate approaches.

At the examination, the horse's head is pushed up into a horizontal position and then brought down again. By doing this, the forward and backward movement of the lower jaw can be assessed in relation to that of the upper jaw. The lower jaw of a normal horse will move back by about 6 to 8 mm in relation to the upper jaw when the head is pushed upward. The incisors clearly show this shift. If there is only a minimum of shift then this can indicate a blocking of the two jaws by, for example, big hooks in front or a step mouth.

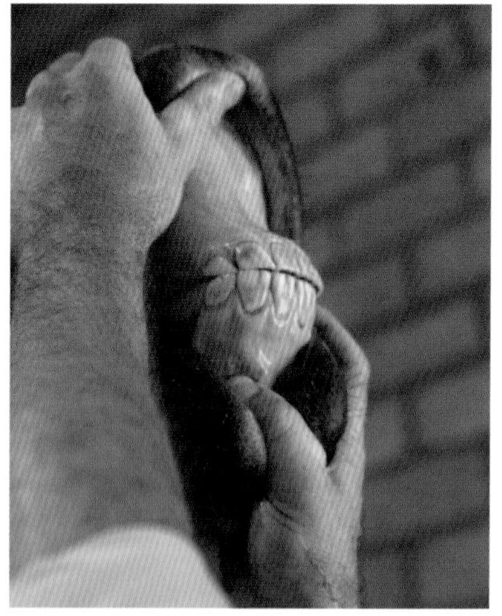

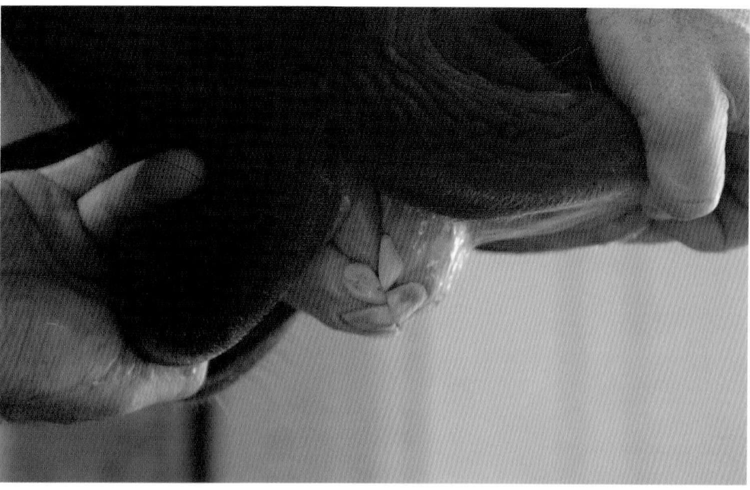

Left and right: The forward and backward mobility of the lower jaw in relation to the upper jaw is checked by pushing the horse's head upward until the teeth are at eye level. The lower incisors will then shift slightly backward in relation to the upper incisors. When the head is brought down to a vertical position again, we normally see the reverse occur. Mobility between 6 to 8 mm is normal.

The sideways movement of the upper and lower jaw in relationship to each other is equally assessed. This is done by pushing the lower jaw sideways in relation to the upper jaw up to the point where an opening is created between the incisors. This normally occurs when the jaw is moved sideways from 1 to 1½ cm. When the upper jaw is pushed to the left, the oblique tables of the right hand molars meet. When it is pushed further sideways, the incisors are pushed further apart. How quickly the incisors can be separated from each other at this moment depends on the angle of the tables of the molars: the maximum sideways divergence in a normal adult horse is about 5 cm. This should be the same on both sides. If this is not the case, it indicates an irregularity of the tables of the molars and perhaps the incisors as well. When the jaw is repeatedly moved to the left and the right, the noise it makes should also be the same. In some horses only a minimal sideways movement is possible and the incisors readily separate and open up high. This immediately indicates that a serious defect of the molars can be expected such as, for example, a shear mouth.

When the lips are opened, the first impression of the incisors is evaluated. They should fit properly together and the tables should form a neat horizontal line when the teeth are viewed at eye level. In the case of uneven incisors, we can also expect problems with the molars due to the sideways movement of the jaws being hindered. If there are injuries on the inside of the lips, check to see whether these are being caused by the incisors having sharp points on the front of the tables, for example. When examining young horses, check for a normal implantation of the incisors and ensure there are no problems with the replacement of the incisors. The age of the animal is estimated and then compared with its actual age. If there appears to be a big discrepancy, then a possible explanation should be sought: occasionally a horse has been sold with the wrong pedigree papers—whether accidentally or deliberately.

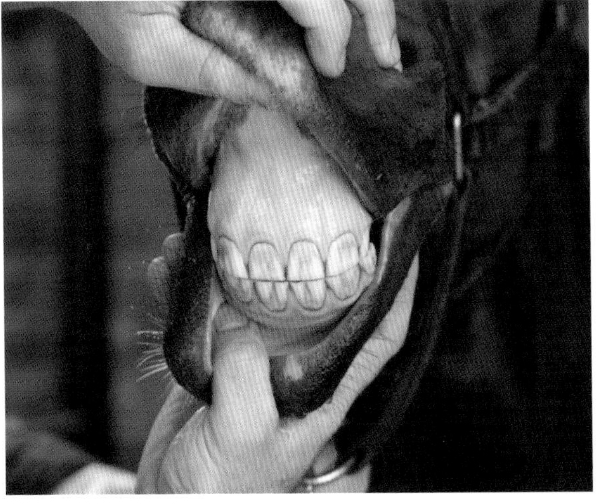
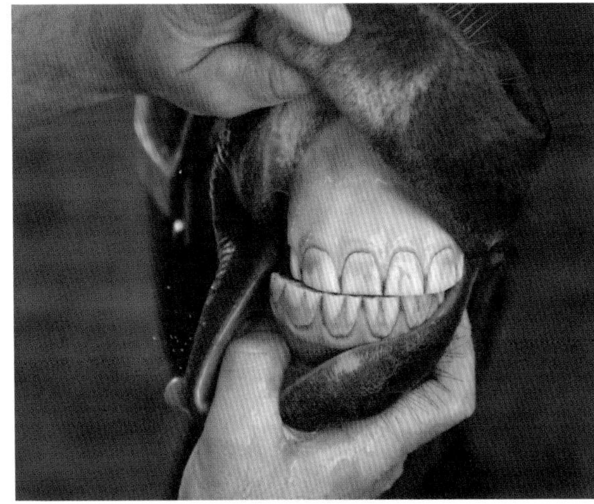
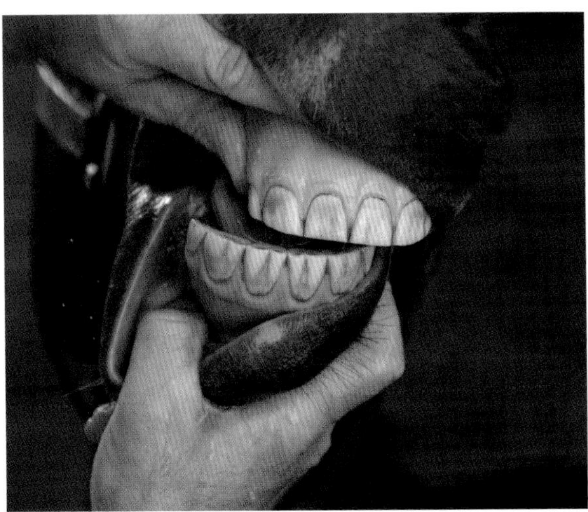
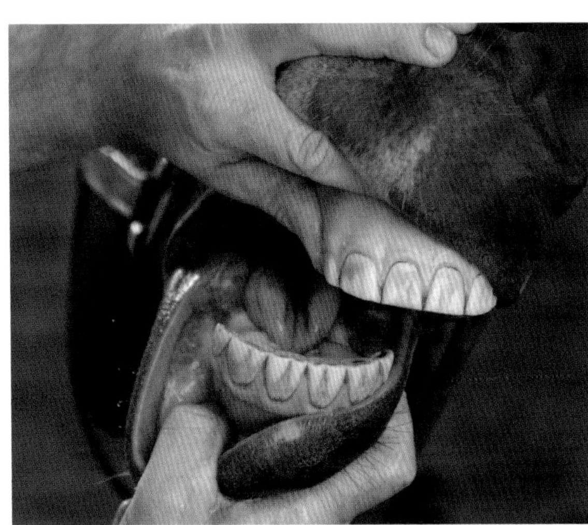

These pictures show the checking of the sideways mobility of the lower jaw in relation to the upper jaw. When there is sideways pressure on both jaws taken in opposite directions, the incisors can be shifted across for about 1 cm before the tables start moving apart. When more sideways pressure is applied, the tables of the incisors move even further away from each other. The maximum sideways movement of an adult horse is about 5 cm and should be nicely symmetrical on both sides of the head.

Examination of the Mouth

Before the mouth can be examined it must first be thoroughly rinsed out to remove any remaining food. A large hand spray of a quarter liter size with an extended opening and a rounded head will ensure that this takes place efficiently and safely. If the mouth is not rinsed then it is often difficult to see small inside cheek injuries among the food remains.

First, the front part of the mouth is inspected. Canines appear in male animals between four to five years of age. The lower canines appear two to eight months earlier than the upper ones. There are one to four rudimentary canines in 25 percent of mares. In older horses I often see plaque on these teeth accompanied by inflammation of the gums.

The point and sides of the tongue are examined for injuries from the incisors or from points on the canines. The upper surface of the tongue is checked for injuries from pressure damage or wounds from the bit. The upper surface of the bars should be level with no swelling or injury caused by the bit.

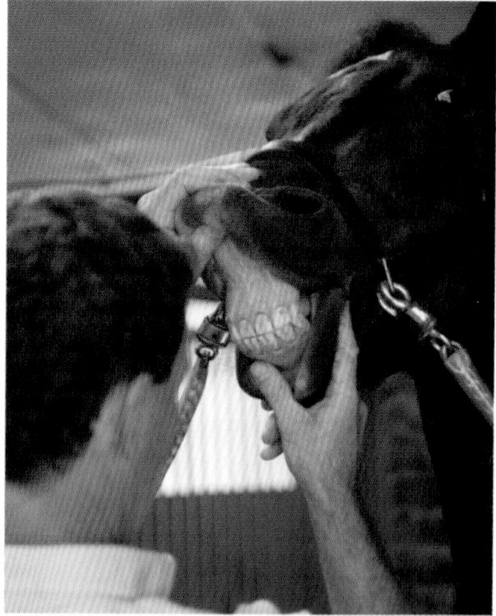

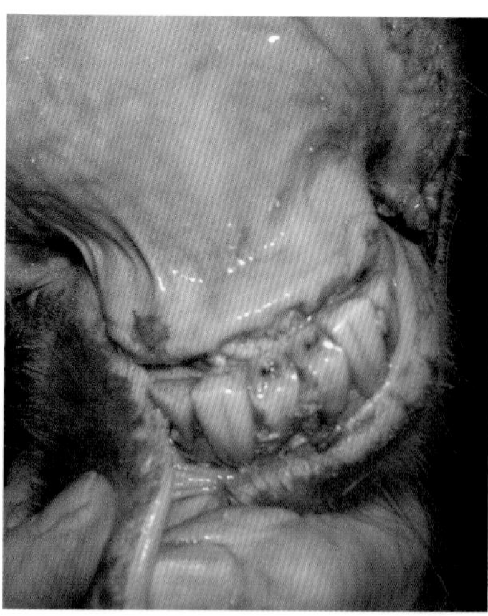

*Top left:
A first impression of the incisors is gained by opening the lips. Normally, the incisors meet together neatly and the tables form a level horizontal line between the incisors.*

*Top right and below:
After opening the lips of this 28-year-old pony it was immediately clear that it must be having difficulties with chewing food. The upper incisors have nearly been completely worn away. The lower incisors are, relatively speaking, much too long and the tables are irregular. This is caused by an inadequate sideways movement of the jaws in relation to each other. This is already an indication that serious dental problems can be expected.*

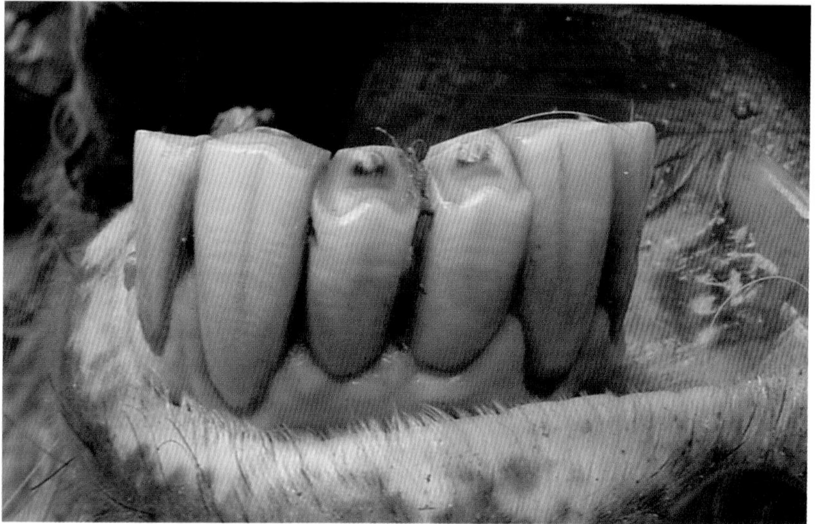

The space in front of the first upper and lower molars is inspected for wolf teeth. Any possible blind wolf teeth can be detected by running the thumb along the edge of the hard palate.

Each molar is felt with the finger tips. Sharp points, raised molars, rear hooks, loose molars and other such defects are detected in this manner. Subsequently, with the aid of a forehead lamp, the molars and the soft mouth tissue are examined for defects. If, despite a mouth rinse, there are still remains of hay caught between the molars these places are more closely examined with a dental mirror. This allows the discovery of diastemas and the degree of the accompanying periodontitis to be assessed. The molars of both the left and right halves of the jaw are checked for symmetry and the angle of the tables is checked.

When examining young animals, there are checks to see whether the arcades of teeth are in good order and whether or not there are any problems with the replacement of the first three molars.

At the end of the examination, the owner is shown any abnormalities in the mouth of the horse. In order for owners to discover, for example,

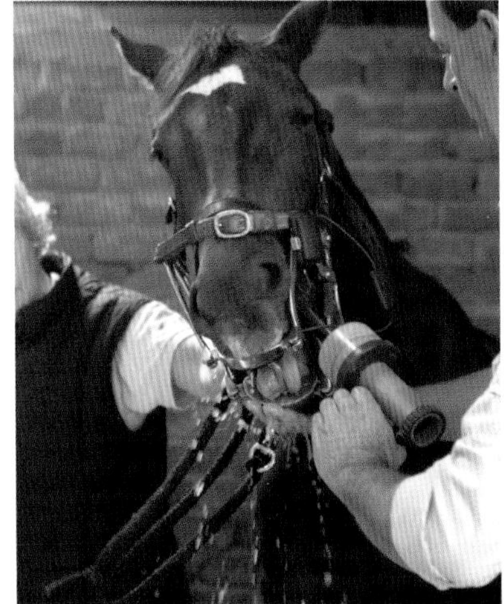

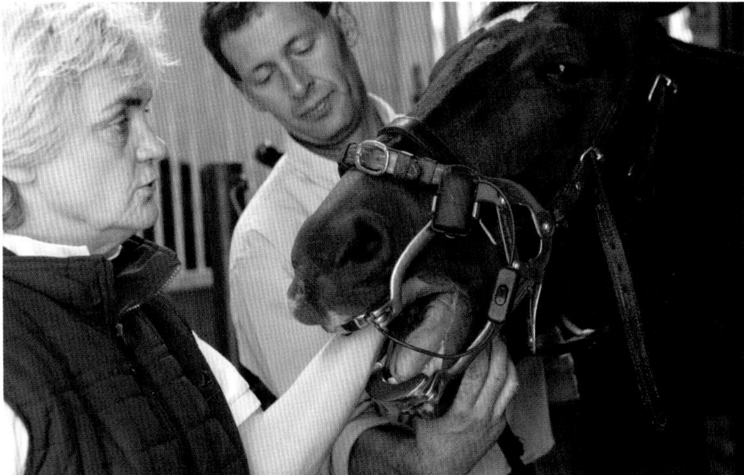

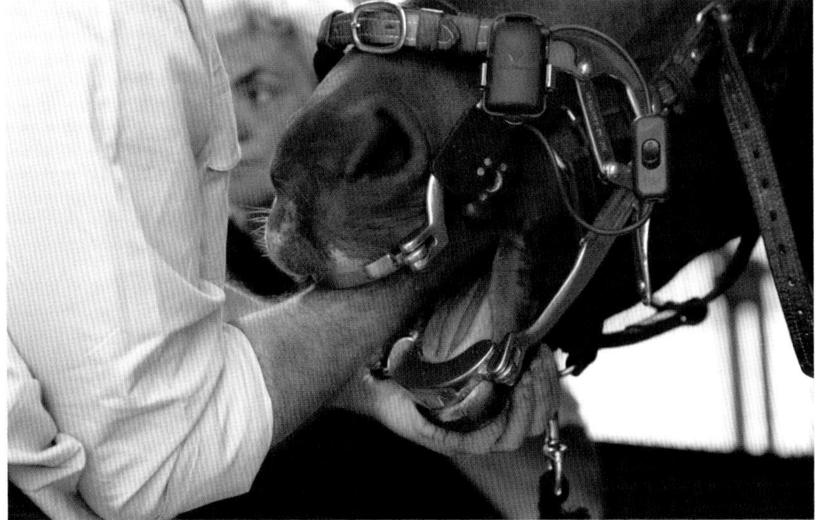

Top left: Before the mouth can be examined, it must first be thoroughly rinsed to remove any remains of food.

Top right:
There is only one way to show owners just how sharp the enamel points of the rearmost molars can be in a horse: let them feel for themselves.

Below:
The examination commences by feeling each of the molars separately. Sharp enamel points, tall molars, loose molars and other defects can be discovered in this way.

just how sharp an enamel point or a rearmost hook can be, there is but one way of finding out: letting them feel it for themselves.

Supplementary Examination Techniques

When a thorough examination of the mouth does not provide a definite diagnosis, there are other valuable methods of examination possible. In cases where there is a suppurating fistula in the jaw bone or sinusitis caused by a bacterial infection of the root of one of the last four upper molars it is sometimes difficult to determine which one of the teeth is causing the trouble. In order to solve the problem, the tooth must be extracted. Seeing that this is a serious intervention for the horse, we turn to supplementary examination techniques to ensure that we can locate the exact tooth.

An extremely familiar examination technique is the taking of X-rays. Due to the great contrast between the density of the structure of the

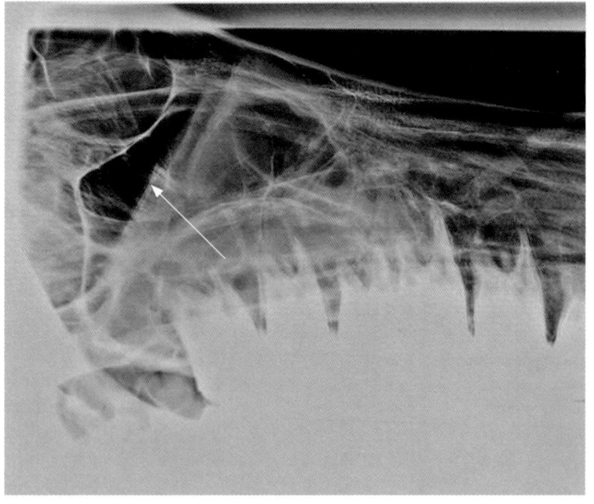

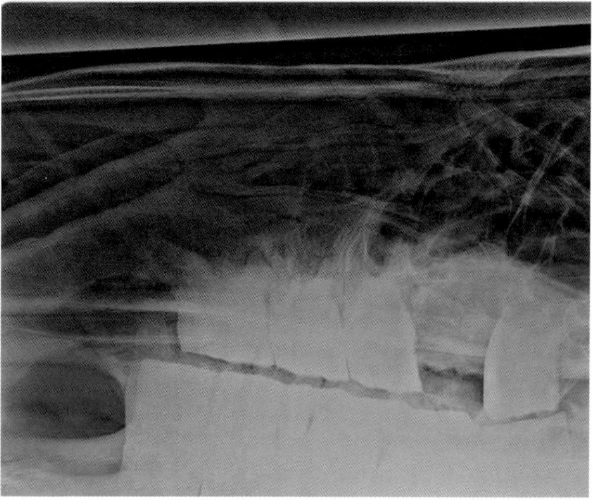

Top left:
The teeth and their roots are clearly seen in an X-ray. This examination however could not identify the tooth that was causing sinusitis in this horse. The fluid line indicates the presence of pus in the sinus cavity.

Top right:
After extraction of a tooth, by way of an X-ray you can check to see if the tooth was removed in its entirety.

teeth and the spaces in the sinuses of the forehead, most equine veterinarians can take good X-rays of horses' teeth. The advantage of this technique is that it can take place while the horse is standing, it is not a complicated method, it is relatively cheap and X-rays can be taken by any veterinarian. They allow the roots of the teeth to be clearly shown. When a fracture in the jaw is suspected, X-rays invariably supply the proof. This technique is also used to detect a root infection and to identify the tooth concerned. Very occasionally this is not successful when using X-rays: in these cases, I wait a couple of weeks until the changes round the dental root concerned have become easier to see or I can switch to using scintigraphy or a CT scan.

In scintigraphy, a radioactive substance is administered to the horse. This radioactive substance is coupled to an element that is continually being built into bone tissue. In the disease process of the bony skeleton, at the level of the injury, there will be an increase of absorption of this element. In the presence of a dental root infection, the surrounding bony tooth socket will also be infected thus showing an increase of absorption. Three hours after being administered, the increased radioactivity is measured on the outside of the head with a sort of Geiger counter (an apparatus that measures radioactive rays). With this sensitive, but expensive technique, it is nearly always possible to detect the tooth concerned. Scintigraphs are only carried out in specialist clinics; indeed, radioactive substances are used and the animals must then spend a night in a separate, secure place. Reading of measurements that are received is also the work of specialists.

A CT scan, or computer tomography is a research method that makes use of X-rays. The permeability of the tissues by these rays is measured by a great number of angles from which the computer then generates a three-dimensional image of the tissue being examined. This technique produces a more detailed image than a simple X-ray and makes it possible to identify even tiny signs of infection round the tooth or in the sinuses of a horse. A possible disadvantage is the need for full anesthesia and the

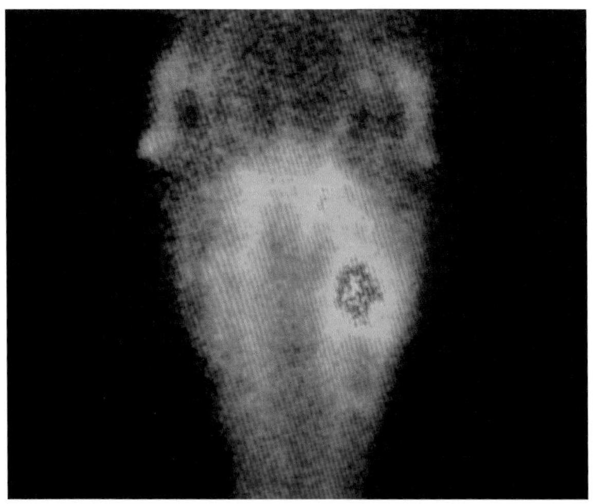

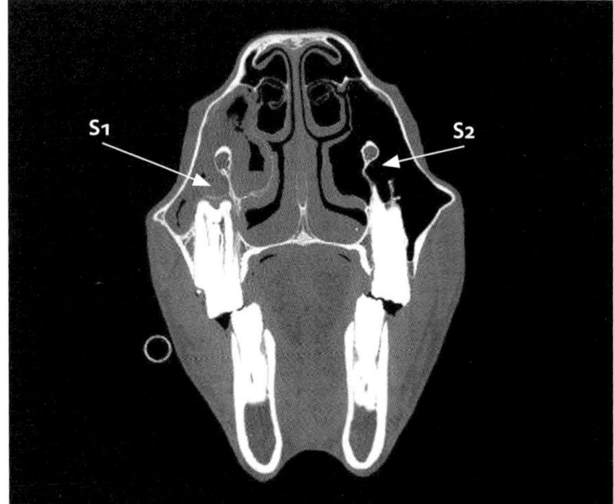

Top left:
The increased absorption of radioactive substance at the level of the molars is seen in this scintigraph image of a horse's head: the horse concerned had sinusitis caused by an infected root. This examination made it clear that the fourth upper molar (209) is the one that must be extracted in order to solve the problem. The "hot spot," that is the red patch with the white center, is exactly at the position of molar 209.

Top right:
A CT scan of a horse with sinusitis. Notice the pus-filled cavity (S1) on the left side. The root of the infected tooth is obviously more rounded than the healthy root on the right side against the empty sinus cavity (S2).

accompanying cost. This technique is only carried out in specialist equine clinics: the performance of the examination and the interpretation of the results is also the work of specialists.

The Dental Record Card

After every examination of the oral cavity a dental record card for the horse is filled in. For reasons of identification this must have the name and address of the owner and an identity for the horse concerned. If there was a specific reason for the requested dental check this is also recorded: then, in follow-up checks, we can ask if problems have been truly resolved. These can be all kinds of issues varying from squirreling food in the cheeks to showing resistance when being ridden to the right. All defects that were observed in the dental examination should be recorded on the card. These can thus be subsequently discussed with the owner. As a result of the findings, a therapy is proposed and an estimate of the costs. The treatment carried out and any medication used is equally recorded. A dental record card facilitates eventual future treatment whether or not by the same dental technician. When there are dental defects, this card identifies special points of interest for the next dental examination. Some defects cannot be corrected in one treatment and a well filled-in card is practically indispensable for the further treatment of such animals.

Frequency of Examinations

Newly born foals are examined for any possible inherited defects such as an overbite. If there are indications for such, it is best to look at them again at around three months. If there is indeed a question of an overbite we can, when it concerns valuable foals, discuss the methods of treatment and put treatment into operation if necessary. The longer such things are

After the dental record card has been filled in, the results of the examination are looked at and the proposed treatment discussed with the owner.

See page 105: A filled-in dental record card

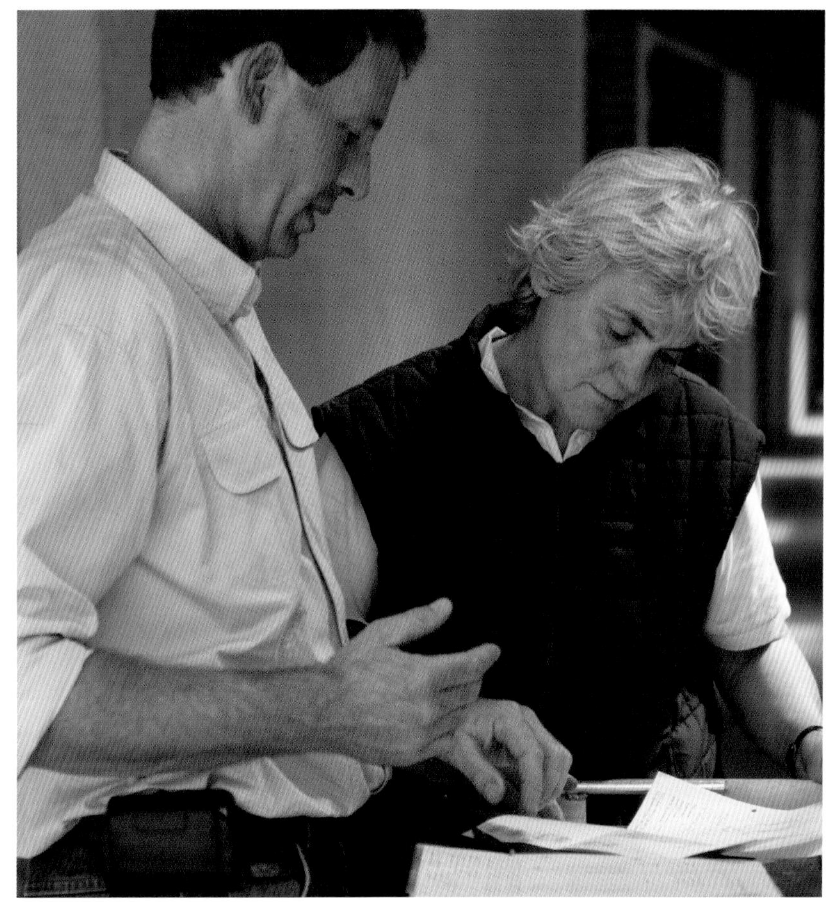

delayed, the smaller the chance of a successful result there will be.

A regular dental check can best be commenced before a young horse is bitted. Indeed, the most active period in the mouth of a horse is between 2½ to 4½ years of age. During this period, a horse loses 24 milk teeth which are replaced with 36 to 44 permanent teeth. Often, the wolf teeth are removed at the first dental examination. During this period, a dental check every half year is advantageous. Three to six months after a cap has been pushed out or removed, the new permanent teeth can already have sharp enamel points. In the period that a horse is being trained it is better that it is not distracted from its work by having pain in its mouth. Some young horses take on bad habits under the influence of these pain sensations: habits that are difficult to eradicate later such as letting its tongue hang out.

A yearly dental check is sufficient for adult horses that are ridden or harnessed regularly. The teeth have all attained their definite place in the mouth. When there are annual checks, not very much can go wrong in the interim period. When there are extensive dental defects, it is usual to plan a separate, individual treatment scheme.

An annual check is usually maintained with senior horses. The chance that problems will arise in the interim period—such as a tooth coming loose—is greater because of the extensive abrasion in older horses. When

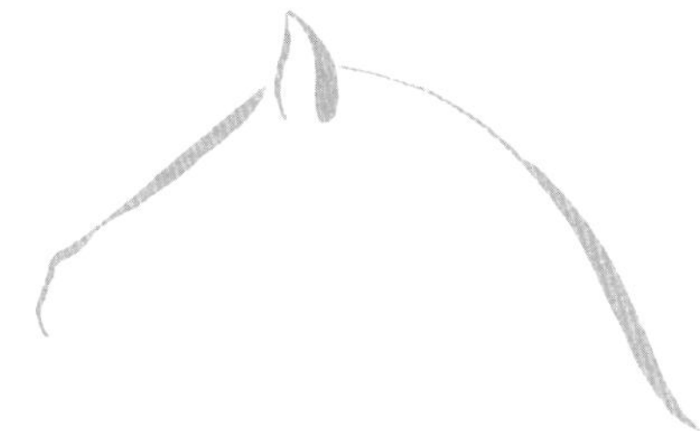

Dr. Chris Hannes

Equine Dental Technician

Owner: Eric Herrygers
Date: 06 / 12 / 07
Address: Congostraat
Horse: Ruben
Katelyne Waver
Type: Warmbloed
Telephone:
Age: 11 y

Remarks: Problemen aanleuning.

Sedation: 0,7 Domosedan
Next Visit: 1 j.

111 110 109 108 107 106 105 104 103 102 101

Above Right
Below Right

311 310 309 308 307 306 304 303 302 301

Above Left
Below Left

111	110	109	108	107	106	105	104	103	102	101	201	202	203	204	205	206	207	208	209	210	211
										gum line											

										gum line											
411	410	409	408	407	406	405	404	403	402	401	301	302	303	304	305	306	307	308	309	310	311

Enamel points: x
Wolf Teeth:
Foremost hook: 2 x
Blind Wolf Teeth:
Rearmost hook:
Caps:

VAT Number: BE 876 914 840

Fortis Bank · Rekening Nr. 001-4685748-45
Iban BE44001468574845 · Bic GEBABEBB

Proosthoevebaan 16 · B-2290 Vorselaar
Telefoon 0479-786.783
info@hanneschris.be
www.hanneschris.be

a horse displays irregularities in its eating pattern, the advice is always to have an interim dental check.

Those against yearly dental checks often present odd arguments: "In the days when horses lived in the wild they didn't have dental checks." Of course, this remark is quite true; it was—and still is—a case of "survival of the fittest" in the wild. In the wild, horses with extensive dental defects lost weight and condition; some of them first succumbed to prey and yet others died an awful death of irreversible weight loss and exhaustion. What is more, horses in the wild did not have a bit in their mouths.

These days we keep our horses for a much longer time, whereas formerly they would have been sent for slaughter. Thus the chance is greater that there will come a time when a horse will have dental problems.

"My parents always kept horses and they never needed to call in a dental technician." This remark is very likely true as well. If a horse was difficult to ride, the first thing that was done was to change to another kind of bit or to have it ridden by a more experienced rider. These horses were often then treated very severely in order to be "corrected." If these measures had no effect, then the horse was often labelled as impossible to ride and sent off to be euthanized. Horses between 15 to 20 years old that had lost too much weight were considered as being prematurely worn out. Actually, it was often only their set of teeth that was prematurely worn out.

CHAPTER 14

Dental Treatment Equipment

Hand Floats

Floats or dental files have been in use for more than 150 years and, to this day, they are still essential and excellent equipment for many dental technicians. Floats consist of a hand grip, a shank, a file top and a rasp. An enormous variation is possible in all these parts.

The type of hand grip depends on the personal choice of the dentist.

The length of the shank depends on which tooth we want to reach in the mouth and what must be done with the tooth. Thus short floats are easier to use when working on the incisors or the first molars. Longer floats are needed for working in the back of the mouth. Some floats have an S-shaped shank for ease of reaching difficult places.

The float head contains the actual rasp. The edges of the float head are rounded to prevent injury to the soft parts of the horse's mouth. Depending on its use, the float head is either a vertical continuation of the shank or it is bent between 5 to 30 degrees upward or downward. Most float heads are so constructed that the rasp itself is easy to replace. The float head and rasp that is made of one piece is thinner, which makes it easier to reach difficult places such as the outside edge of the table of the last upper molar. However, the disadvantage of these hand floats is that when the rasping surface is no longer sharp—and can no longer be sharpened—they have to be replaced in their entirety.

The rasp itself consists of an extremely tough metal alloy. Depending on the manufacturer, there are usually three grades of coarseness of the rasp surface: fine, medium and coarse. The first two are usually used for

Below left:
The length and form of the shank of the float depends upon which tooth is being treated and its position in the mouth.

Below right:
Depending on what has to be done with a specific tooth, the float head is situated on the shank at a certain angle, either upward or downward.

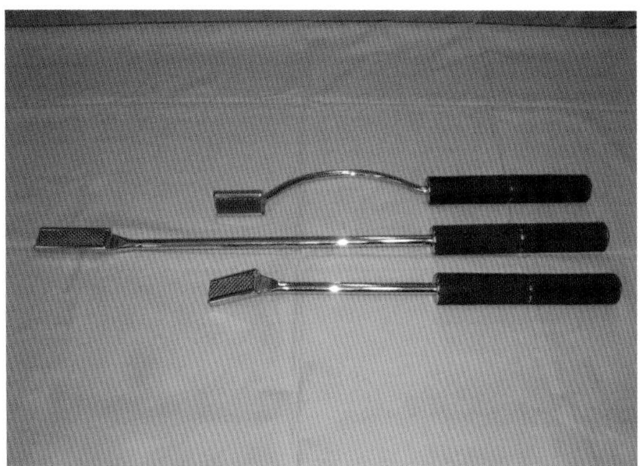

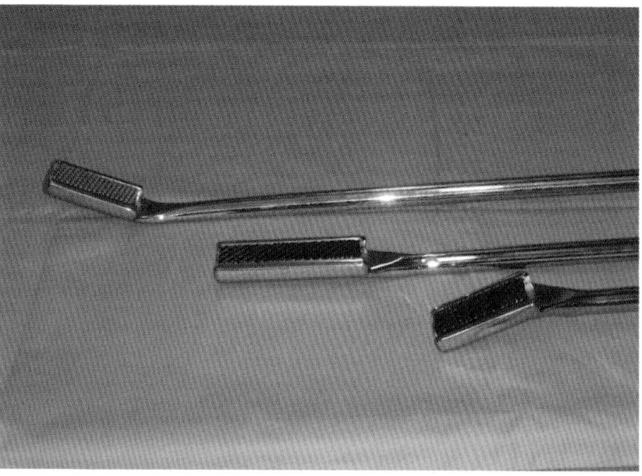

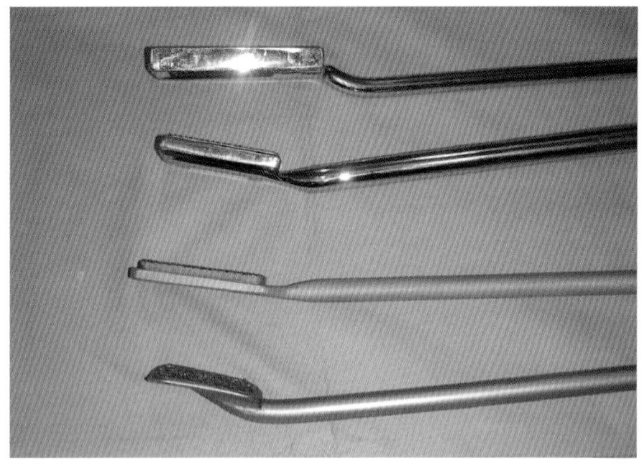

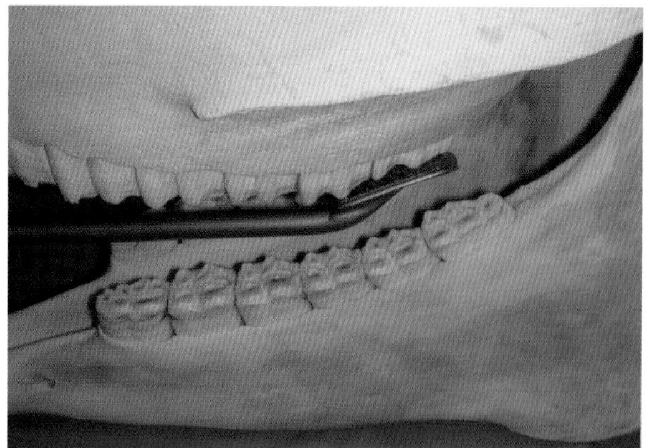

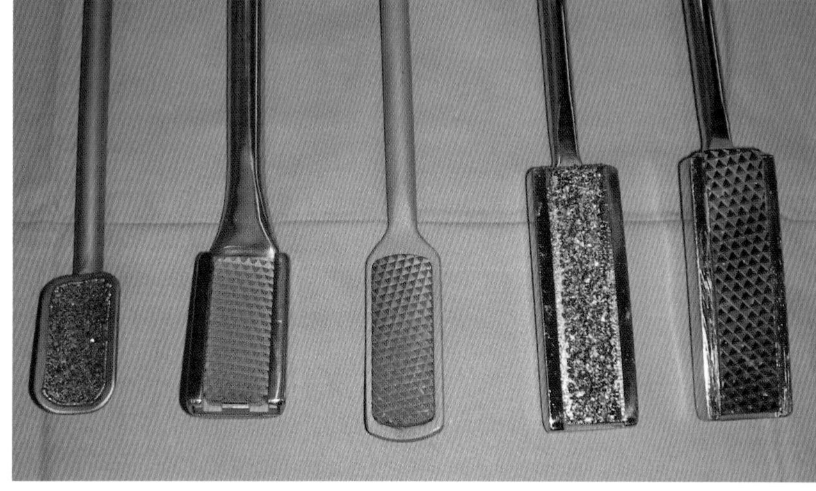

Top left:
The float heads themselves come in various thicknesses. For places difficult to reach such as the outside of the last upper molar, it is an advantage to have a float head that is as thin as possible.

Top right:
This is the ideal hand float for the last upper molar. The float is long enough to reach the tooth, the float head is lightly angled upward like the tables of the molars and the float head itself is extremely thin because the diamond particles are set directly on the head.

Below:
The left hand float head is set with industrial diamonds. The other four rasps are composed of various metal alloys. The composition determines the hardness of each rasp and the length of use.

preventive work. The coarse version is used for filing away large parts of the tooth such as the foremost hook. These floats become less and less sharp with use and must be regularly replaced. In recent years, hand floats with a diamond layer on the float head have also become available. These float heads remain sharp for a long time and because they are less thick they are very good for reaching difficult places.

In general, the dental technician will have a wide selection of various hand floats among his equipment. They will be used interchangeably depending on the mouth and the desired result. It is not possible to maintain a horse's set of teeth properly with only a couple of hand floats.

Electrical Apparatus

In the last ten years, a lot more use has been made of power floats. Depending upon the movement of the rasp blade, these floats can be divided into three groups: the rasp blade can be moved on a horizontal plane backward and forward; the rasp head is cylindrical and turns on its own axis; the rasp head is circular and turns on the horizontal plane on the rasp shank. The rasp itself mostly consists of a hard metal alloy or

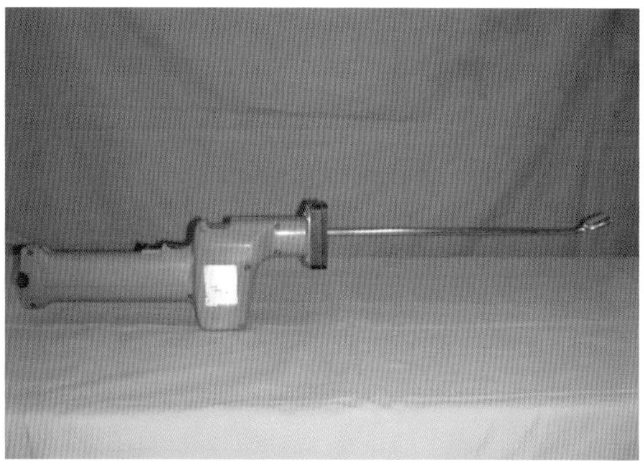

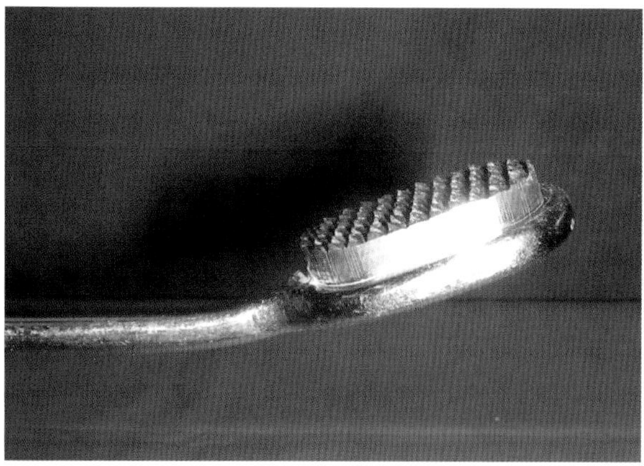

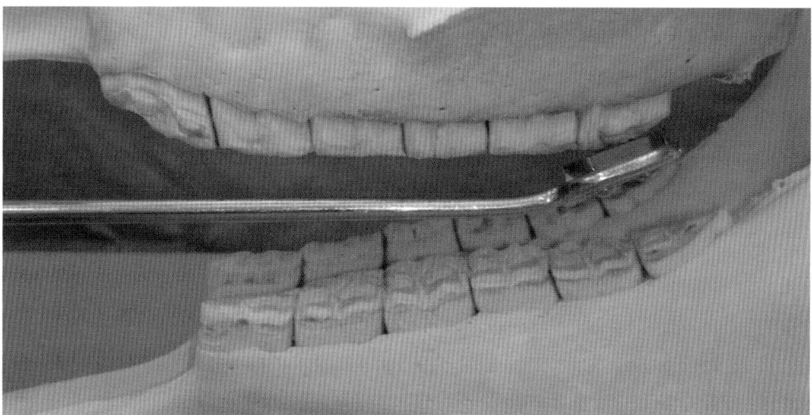

Top three pictures:
The first type of power float has a rasp head that moves automatically back and forth in a way similar to a hand float. The number of movements (up to 1000 per minute) is far more than that of a hand float—the speed of work is tremendously improved. The rasp head itself is often composed of the same metal alloy used in hand floats.

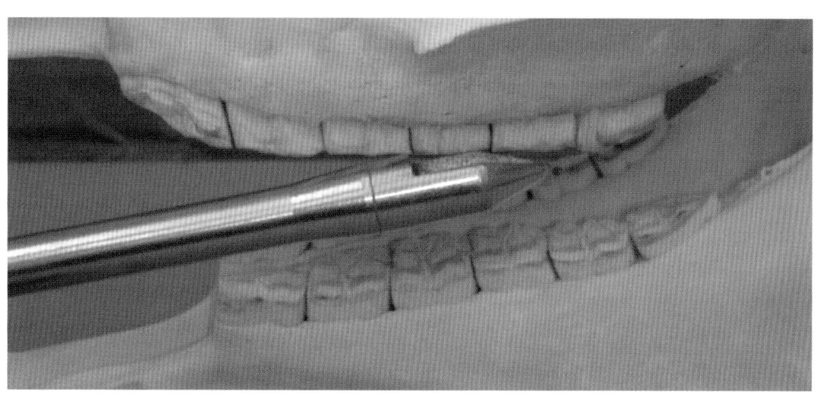

Bottom three pictures:
The second type of power float has a cylindrical rasp head that turns on its own axis. These floats are often set with industrial diamonds.

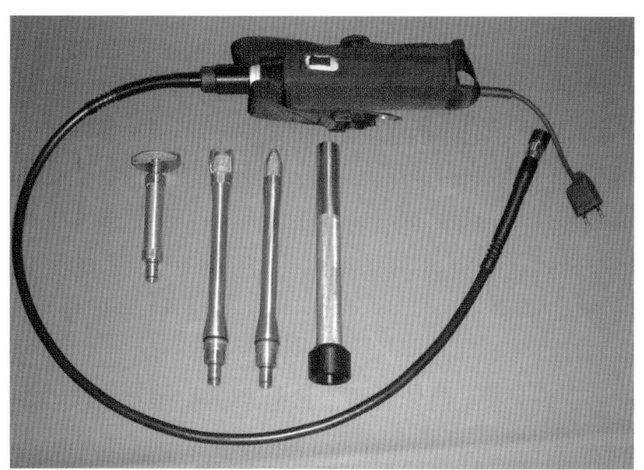

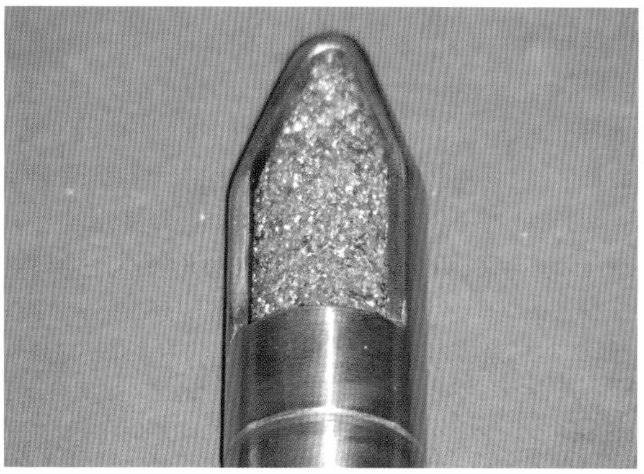

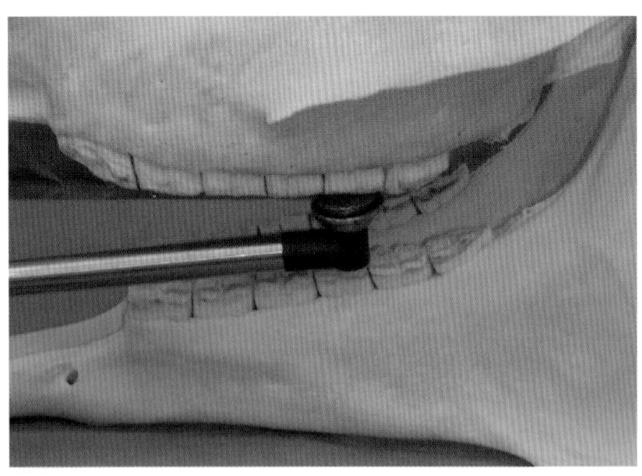

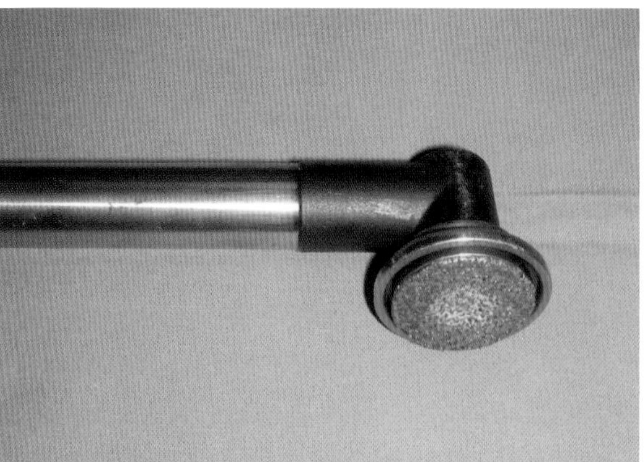

All three pictures: This type of power float has a circular rasp head and turns on the same plane as the rasp shank.

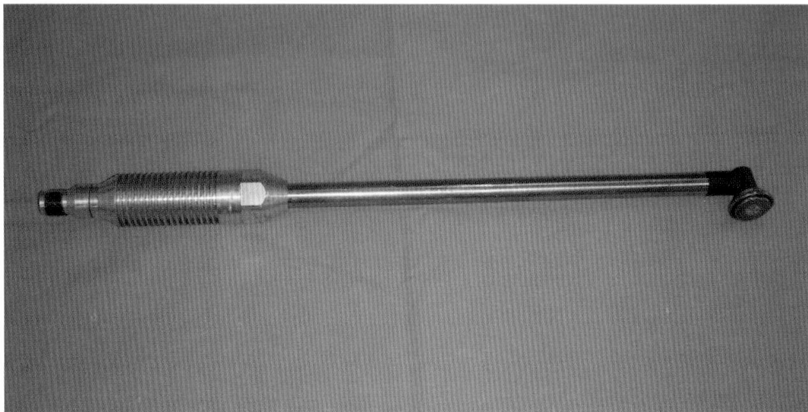

it has an industrial diamond covering. On the upper part and sides the rasp is protected so that no delicate parts of the mouth can be injured. These floats can easily be used in normal treatment but above all they are useful when extensive corrections have to be made such as reducing teeth that are too long.

Here too, various rasp heads are available depending on the place in the mouth that needs to be worked on.

The use of electrical equipment is sometimes questioned. Opponents claim that the speed of this type of float limits the tooth life by filing down the table unnecessarily. In normal care of the teeth, there is seldom a need to file down the tables of the teeth. The advantage of this equipment is its speed: floating the whole surface of a tooth that is too long can be done much more efficiently. The treatment time is also much shorter for the horse. In combination with a good source of light, these floats can be used efficiently and safely. In the hands of an inexperienced person they can, of course, be a danger to your horse but this would also be the case with hand floats.

Electrical equipment causes higher friction, which brings with it the chance of the tooth becoming overheated. When extensive corrections are called for it is best to cool the mouth by rinsing at intervals and cooling the rasp head by plunging it in water.

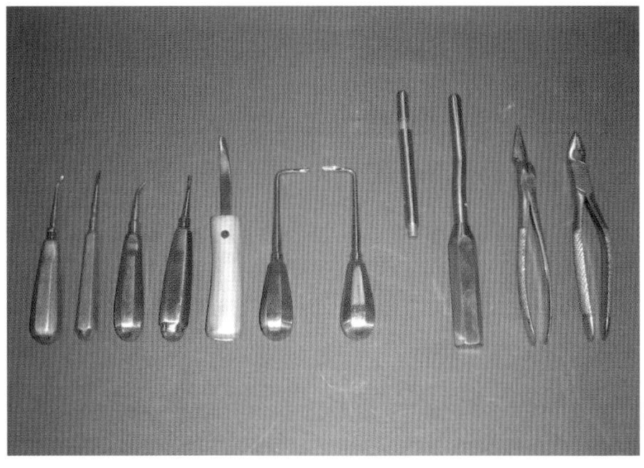

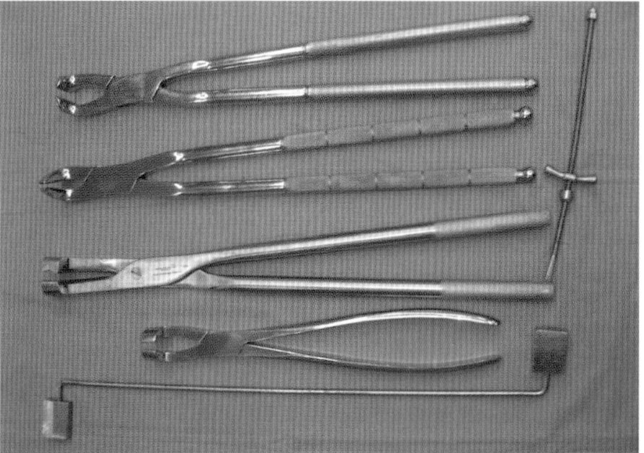

Extraction Equipment

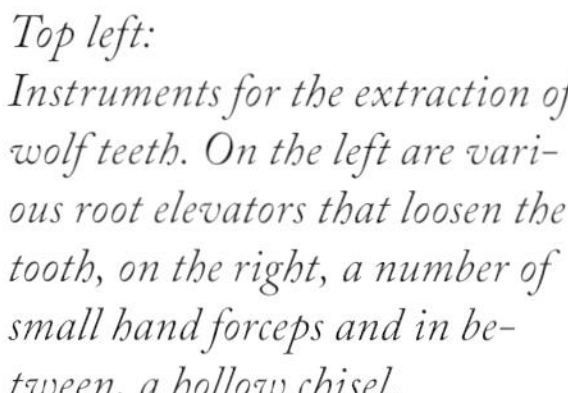

Top left:
Instruments for the extraction of wolf teeth. On the left are various root elevators that loosen the tooth, on the right, a number of small hand forceps and in between, a hollow chisel.

Top right:
Instruments for the extraction of molars. On the bottom is a fulcrum or support, above this are three molar forceps, and at the top, a molar separator.

Wolf teeth are often extracted early on in a horse's sport career. For this, all sorts of small hand instruments have been developed. The selection of root extractors or elevators is extremely broad and depends on the personal choice of the dental technician. Sometimes a hollow, cylindrically formed chisel is pressed over the wolf tooth that cuts into the surrounding gums. The point of the root extractor can be placed in this groove in order to further loosen the root. However, if the hollow chisel is used to extract the tooth, it nearly always results in a broken-off wolf tooth. Small extraction forceps are used to pull the loose wolf tooth from its socket.

The instruments for extracting molars are of quite another order. With these, work must often take place right in the back of the mouth. A molar spreader has a wedge-shaped head that is very gradually closed down on the front and back of the molar to be extracted. The buildup of pressure gradually tears loose the fibers by which the dental cementum is anchored into the socket. The head of the long molar forceps should neatly fit round the crown of the tooth in order to apply the necessary force without the forceps slipping from the tooth. A fulcrum or support is placed between the tooth in front and the forceps handles. In this way the long handles act as a lever to work the tooth in question free from the arcade of teeth.

Below left and right:
A molar separator has a wedge-shaped head that is slowly worked between the teeth to break the attachment from the socket at the front and back of the tooth to be extracted.

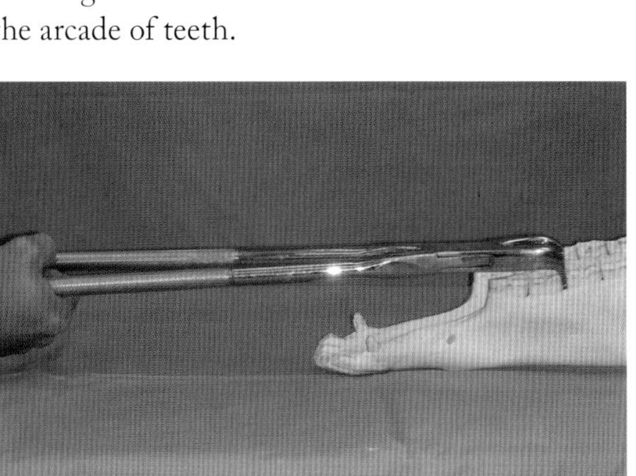

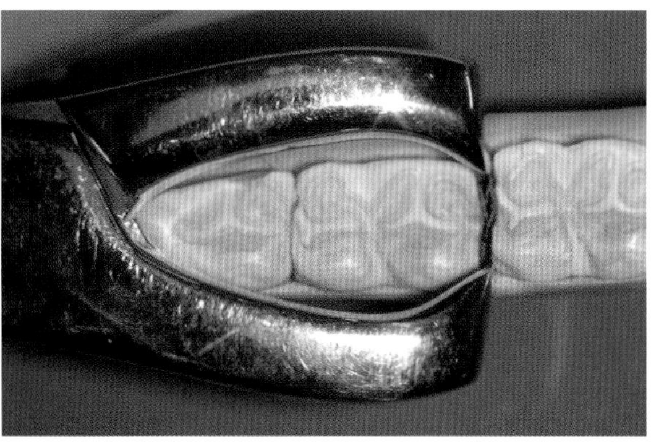

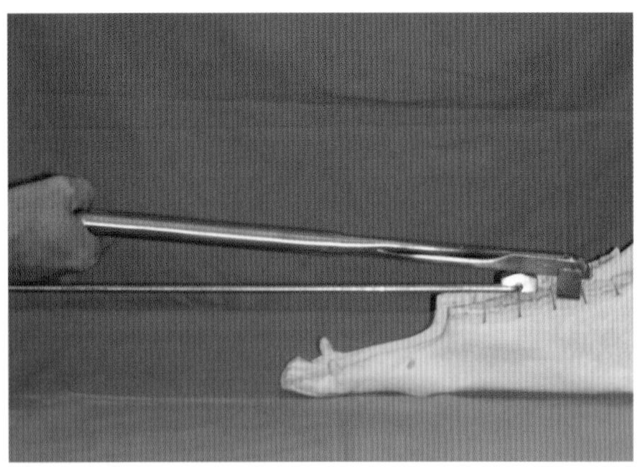

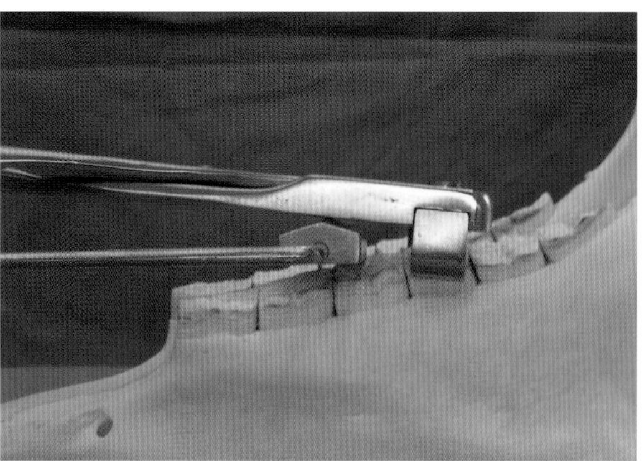

Top left and right: The molar is gradually worked loose from the socket with the large molar forceps. When the tooth is loosened enough, a fulcrum is placed under the molar forceps so that a lever action can be created in order to extract the tooth.

For the extraction of persistent milk incisors, frequently the same elevators or forceps are used as those for wolf teeth. For the removal of caps, an adapted short molar forceps is used: the caps forceps.

Formerly, large molar clippers or a gouge were used to reduce elevated molars or their parts. The elevated part could be properly removed in this way but the risk that the rest of the crown and root would break was always present. The development of the power float has made these instruments redundant today.

CHAPTER 15

The Dental Treatment

There are two important reasons for having dental treatment, the most frequent one being in order to make the horse's mouth comfortable for wearing a bit. A horse with pain in the mouth cannot accept the bit well, and will show resistance more often. The second reason is to improve the chewing function of the molars so there can be better grinding and exploitation of food.

There are two ways in which the dental treatment can be carried out on a horse in a standing position. The first way is by "feel": here, the horse's head is at the chest height of the dental technician and floating is done by feel. At intervals, the situation is monitored by hand palpation or by shining a light in the mouth. The advantage of this method is—usually—the horse does not need to be anesthetized. When a horse has a normal set of teeth that only need minor corrections, this is a very serviceable method. When there are many corrections needed or if there are major defects such as a tall molar, then the above method often leads to an unsatisfactory result.

The second way of working is "under visual control." Here, the horse's opened mouth is held at the eye level of the dental technician. This is best

Left:
One way of floating is by "feel." The horse's head is placed at chest height to the dental technician and the float is used by feel in the horse's mouth. This is the usual method for minor corrections of the teeth.

Right:
Another way of working is under "visual control." At every stage of the treatment there is visual control from the continuous use of a source of light; here it is fixed to the back of the upper incisors. This method allows more accurate work to be done.

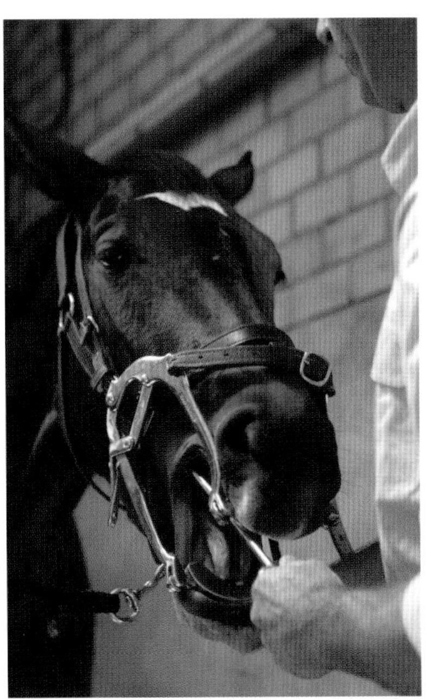

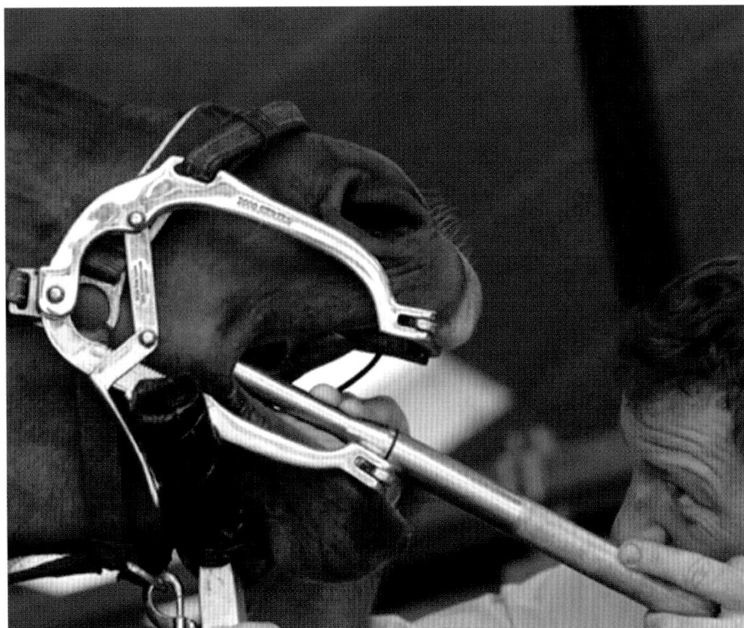

achieved by using a head support or a dental stand. The horses that are treated in this way are put under anesthetic. Due to the continuous use of a light source, there is time for inspection at every stage of the treatment. The instruments can be accurately placed and the discomfort to the horse kept to a minimum. Major corrections can also be carried out more speedily. Some procedures are very difficult—even impossible—to carry out without this method, for example, tooth extraction or removing food remains from diastemas.

The use of anesthetics for dental treatment is still controversial. Some technicians even proudly announce the fact that they can treat a horse without resorting to anesthetics—as if this was the most important goal of dental treatment! Internationally, it is becoming more and more accepted that it is not possible to give a thorough dental treatment without anesthetics. Considering the limited space in the mouth it is not impossible to imagine that a file can sometimes touch the wrong spot. If, at that moment, the horse also shakes its head or makes a defensive move, it doesn't take much for it to turn into a very unpleasant experience. At times like this, often treatment has to be stopped—not because it is finished but because the horse shows more and more resistance.

All too often I see horses that have been treated but where the outer edge of the upper molars still have enamel points with the accompanying injury to the inside of the cheeks. A hook at the back of the last lower molar is also often left untreated. Due to the nearness of the entrance to the throat, horses find a correction at this spot unpleasant. It is quite unacceptable for a dental technician to boast that anesthetics will not be used and then leave such things unattended.

The advantages of the use of an anesthetic are legion. It makes the dental treatment much safer for the owner and the dental technician. The owner does not have to worry beforehand about holding the horse for the technician or be concerned that the horse will undergo an unpleasant experience. However, the most important advantage is that the proposed treatment can be carried out in a comfortable and careful way.

These days, there are sedatives that have been specifically developed for horses. Depending on the dose and the type of sedative, horses can be sedated for 30 minutes to two hours. Some horses begin to sweat lightly during this period; this is only a temporary symptom. There is no contraindication for use of these sedatives for mares in foal. However, we do know that their use at the end of the pregnancy causes a heightened activity in the smooth muscle cells of the wall of the womb. It is for this reason, as a precaution, that mares are not sedated in the last three months of their pregnancy. It is a good idea to take this fact into account when planning dental treatment for broodmares.

In dental care we can differentiate between various treatments to be carried out. These will be examined below with their separate treatment protocol:

- Preventive dental care
- Dental care for horses being ridden or harnessed
- Correction of major dental defects
- Extraction of teeth

Preventive Dental Care

A sacred principle in medicine for both man and beast is "prevention is better than cure." Possible causes of the progress of an illness can be removed in time in horses that show no external symptoms of a disorder. In the treatment of teeth we can take as examples the removal of enamel points, which cause injury to the inside of the cheeks or to the tongue, and the correction of minor defects.

Pain changes the chewing mechanism. Ultimately, this causes abnormal abrasion of the tables, which in turn leads to the development

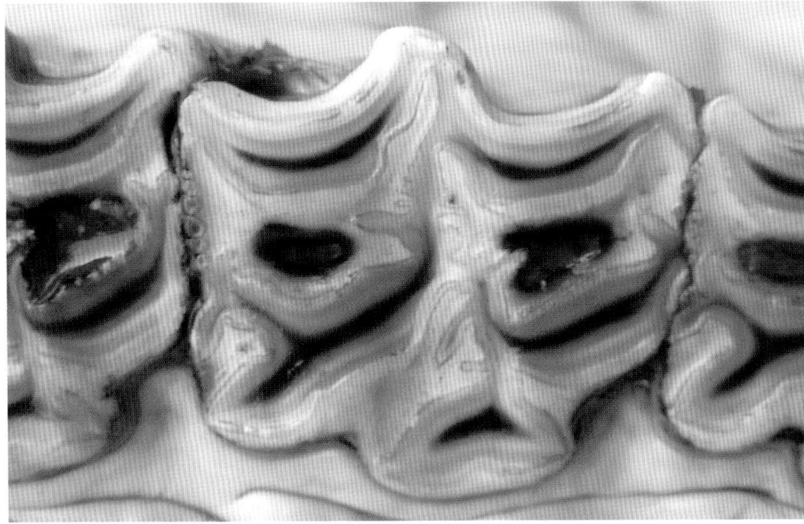

Top and below left:
The sharpness of the enamel points is determined by the construction of the molar. In the top picture, the undulations on the outer edge of the table of the molar are far more extreme than those in the picture below left. Relatively speaking, the enamel points protrude much further from the side surface of the molar; they are more likely to cause injury to the inside of the cheek.

Below right:
The inside cheek injuries are caused by sharp enamel points on the outer edge of the upper molars. These are seen all too frequently in horses that are ridden or harnessed. How can we ever say such horses have a "comfortable" mouth?

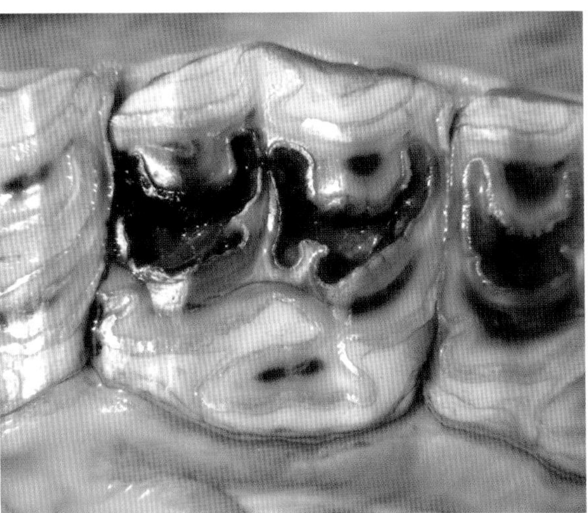

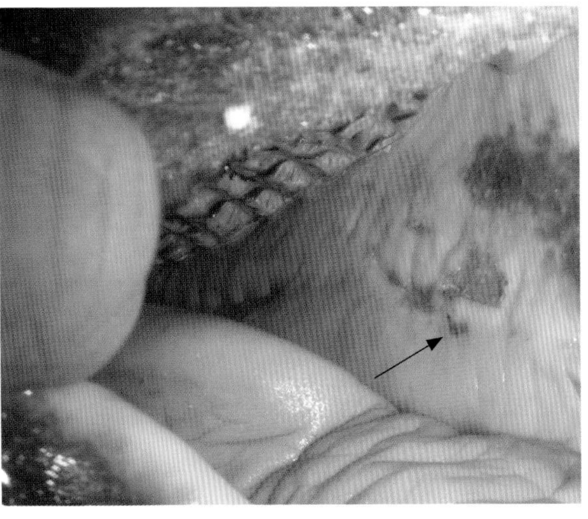

Top left and right:
The outside edge of the tables of the upper molars and the inside edge of the tables of the lower molars are floated to remove the sharp enamel points.

Below left:
The protruding enamel points are clearly observable on the cheek side: they have caused injury to the cheek.

Below right:
After floating, the enamel points have been removed and the outer edge of the table has been nicely smoothed. Comfort in the mouth of this horse has been considerably improved.

of greater dental defects such as shear mouth. The horse then enters a vicious circle: the chewing mechanism becomes even more unbalanced and the dental defects become even more serious. This finally results in the inability to take in sufficient food and the horse loses weight. In the end, this can lead to the horse's death.

Older horses often die because they cannot grind their food finely enough and they become very weak. In this way, they are, of course, vulnerable to all kinds of other conditions. People often say that an old, thin horse is "finished" but it is mostly a case of just the teeth being "finished": unhappily, the rest of the horse will follow.

Therefore, the floating of enamel points forms the basis of every dental treatment. The outside edge of the upper molars and the inside edge of the lower molars are filed down. Enamel points are removed: they are properly smoothed down where they come into contact with the tongue and the cheeks. This prevents the development of painful wounds caused by the enamel points during the chewing process. Due to the abrasion

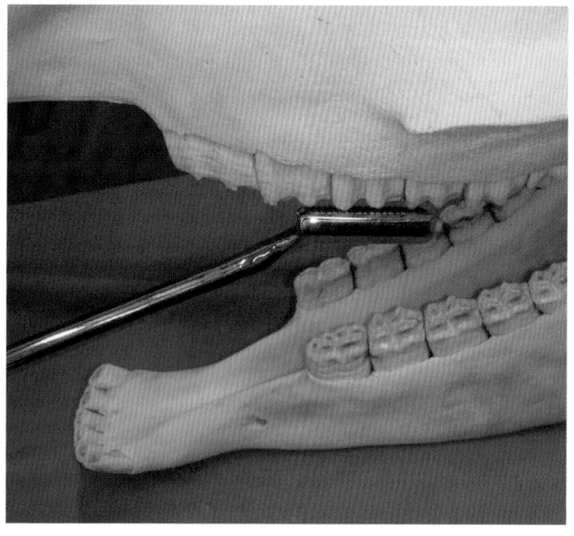

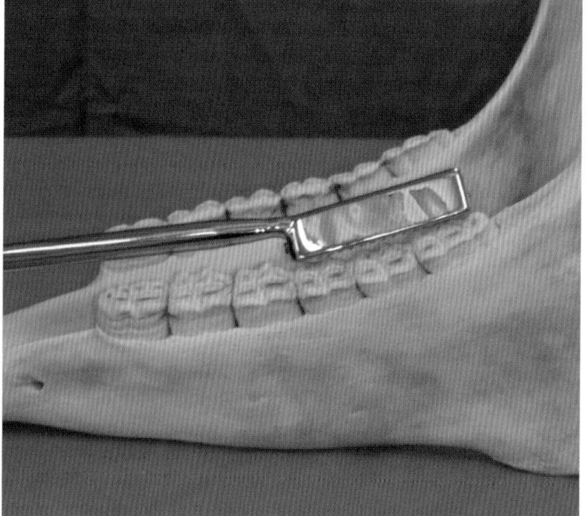

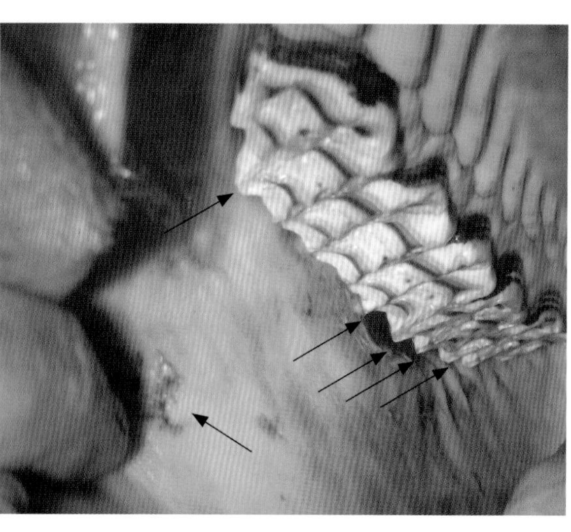

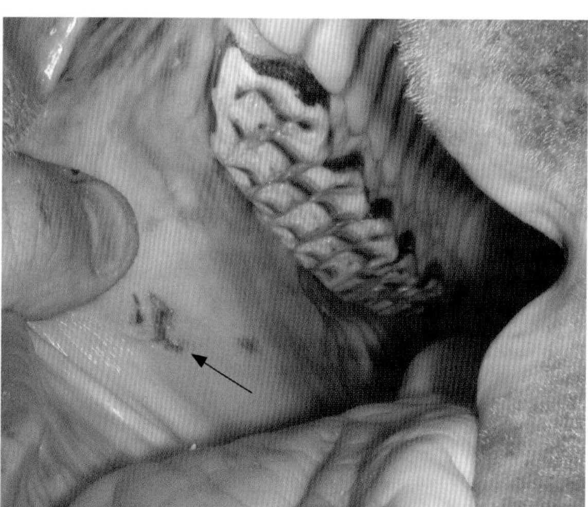

of the molar tables (about 2 to 3 mm per year) these enamel points will repeatedly develop because, once the tables have worn down again below the rounding off, new enamel points start to arise. The yearly dental checkup is based on the rate of development of the new enamel points.

Floating is meant to remove the sharp enamel points from the edge of the table: it is not meant to rasp the table completely smooth. The undulating enamel on the table surface is indeed what allows the horse to more effectively chew its food. If this surface is completely filed down, the horse will not be able to extract energy from its food during the next six weeks due to a poor grinding mechanism. After this period, the softer dentine and the cementum are worn down further than the hard enamel and the table surface is once again able to operate more efficiently. A horse with properly floated teeth has had the tables disturbed as little as possible.

The 11 to 13 usual transverse ridges on the tables of an arcade of molars are natural phenomena. When the horse is being ridden, they do not hinder the forward and backward motion of the lower jaw: it is only during eating that the molars actually come together with the help of the big chewing muscles. When the horse's chewing muscles are not in use, there is a small free space between the molars—just as there is in humans. It is only when these transverse ridges are bigger than a few millimeters—thus much too long—that they may be reduced in height. Some dental technicians make it their business to float the molars until they are smooth—consequently going against the evolution of horses' teeth over the centuries. "Nicer" is certainly not "better" for your horse—on the contrary.

Dental Care for Riding and Driving Horses

The aim here is to provide the horse with as much comfort in the mouth as possible when a bit is being used. The usual place for the bit for most horses is a couple of centimeters in front of the first molars. Normally the bit rests on top of the tongue. With the ideal horse and perfect contact—contact without pressure on one's hands—the bit stays beautifully in position at this place.

However, this ideal is usually only something that we can dream about. Most horses are far from having perfect light contact and most riders have too much weight in their hands. It is thus that the bit is frequently pulled from its ideal place and painful situations can develop. If the horse pokes its nose in front, the bit is pulled toward the first molars. The lip creases on the inside of the corners of the mouth can then become caught between the bit and the first molars. This can cause small bruises or wounds on the inside of the corners of the mouth.

If there are upper or lower wolf teeth just in front of the first molars, the bit can strike against them. It is because of the small size of the wolf teeth that this interference can cause a slight traction on the fibers that anchor the tooth in the socket in the mouth. It is very likely that the horse finds the tapping of the metal bit against the tiny tooth extremely unpleasant (just try tapping the handle of a soup spoon against your own teeth!). If the crown of the wolf tooth is very pointed it can cause injury to the corners of the mouth.

These sensations of pain can upset a horse in its work and does not allow it to give its best performance. When making a turn on the haunches, a little bit of resistance can cause a dressage horse to suddenly press its back leg into the ground instead of lightly lifting it on the beat as it should. With show jumping horses, a little bit of resistance can have grave consequences if it is in the middle of a triple bar jump. More information concerning this can be found in the chapter called "The importance of a bit that fits properly" on page 131.

As has previously been described here, the removal of enamel points is the first requirement for a comfortable mouth.

Every horse that regularly uses a bit can benefit from a "bit seat." This involves the front side of the first upper and lower molars being smoothly rounded—just like the top of one's finger. If the rider pulls on the reins, the inside of the corners of the mouth come against these smoothly rounded molars. In this way, there will be no more injuries to the inside corners of the mouth.

Below left and right: The white, transparent sharp enamel points on the outer edge of the first molar (left) were filed away and the front of the molars were smoothly rounded (right). This is the basic treatment for all horses wearing a bit in their mouths.

The wolf teeth and blind wolf teeth are often removed in young sport horses because they can cause bit discomfort. Before extraction, the gums surrounding the wolf tooth are made numb by local anesthetic. From an animal welfare standpoint, it is indefensible to loosen and extract these teeth without administering an anesthetic. Just imagine if your own dentist did such a thing. Nevertheless, this often happens with horses:

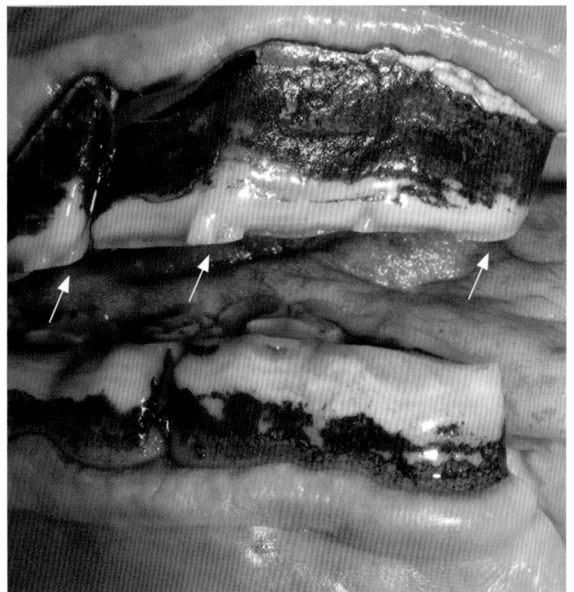

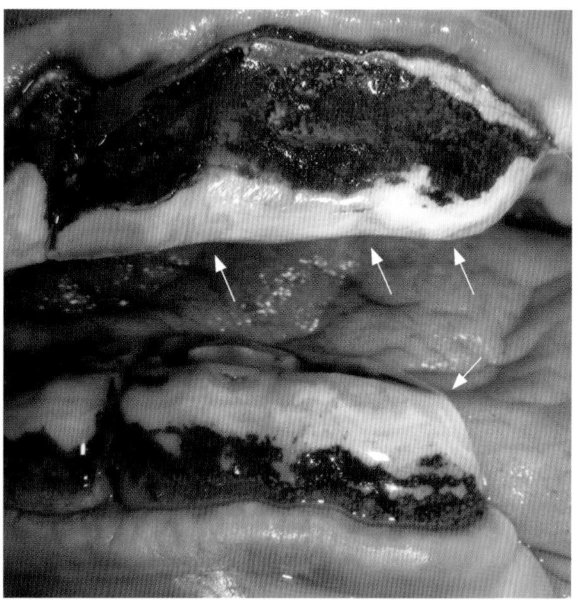

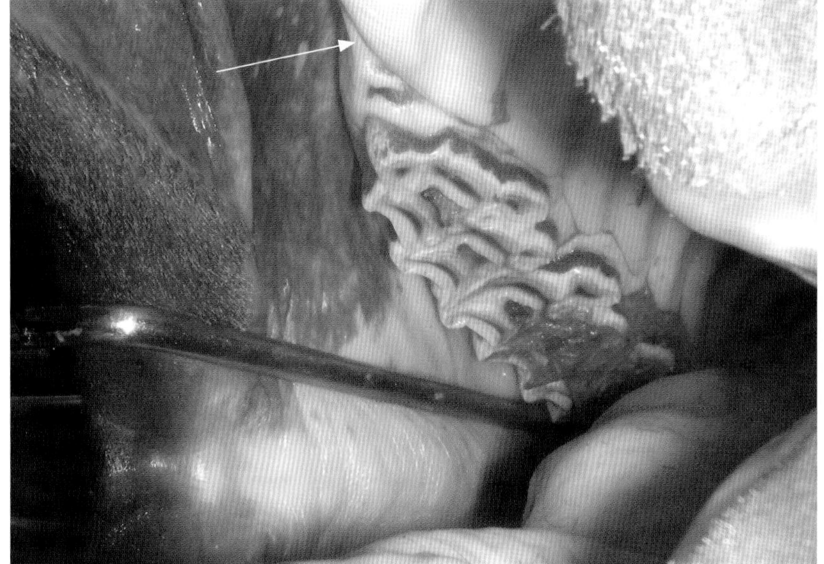

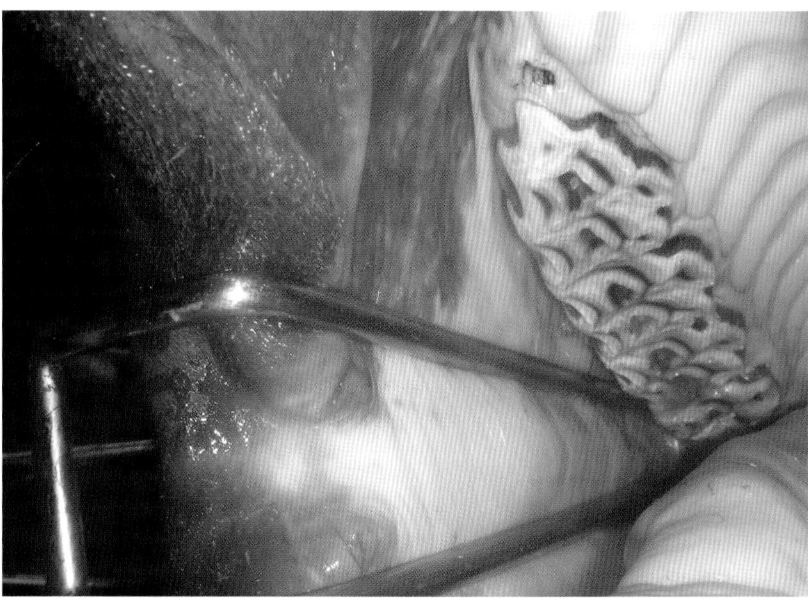

Top:
This horse had problems working on the bit: it displays the root of a wolf tooth that has broken off just under the level of the gums. Bit pressure presses the surrounding gums into the sharp remains of the root.

Below:
After removal of the remains of the wolf tooth, the horse was made much more comfortable when being ridden.

a hollow chisel is placed over the crown of the wolf tooth and, with one movement, the chisel is pressed into the gums and the tooth twisted out. Often, the horse reacts to the sudden pain with the result that there is frequently a broken-off wolf tooth instead of an extracted one. This technique seldom, in fact, results in a completely removed wolf tooth. If the break in the root occurs deep enough in the socket, it usually does not cause further problems. However, when the resulting serrated line of the fracture is just under the gums, it is at this point that the sharp edges will be pressed into the gums when there is pressure from the bit. These broken-off wolf teeth will then be the cause of even more problems than previously encountered.

When the horse is sedated and a local anesthetic has also been ad-

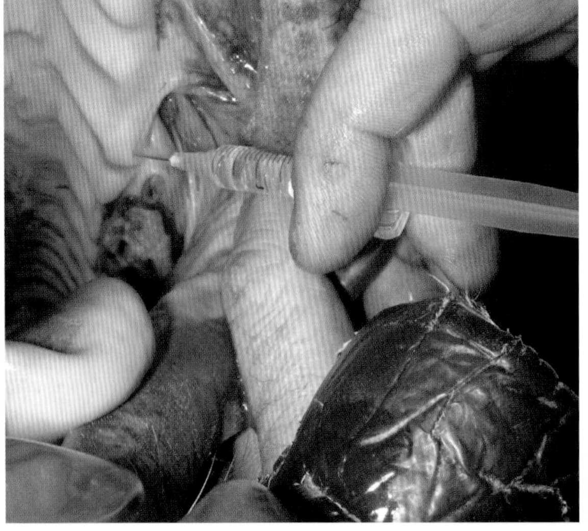

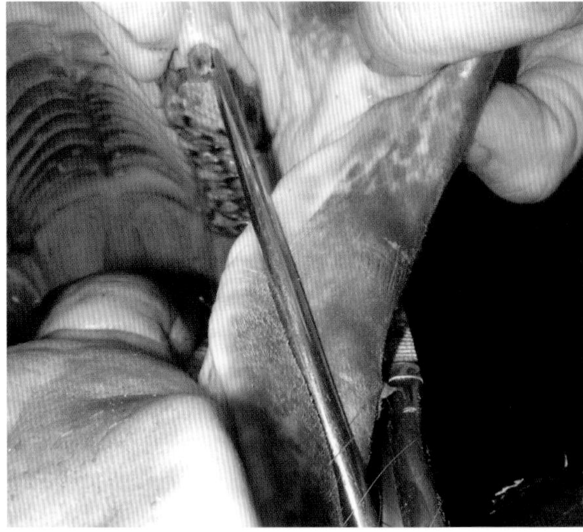

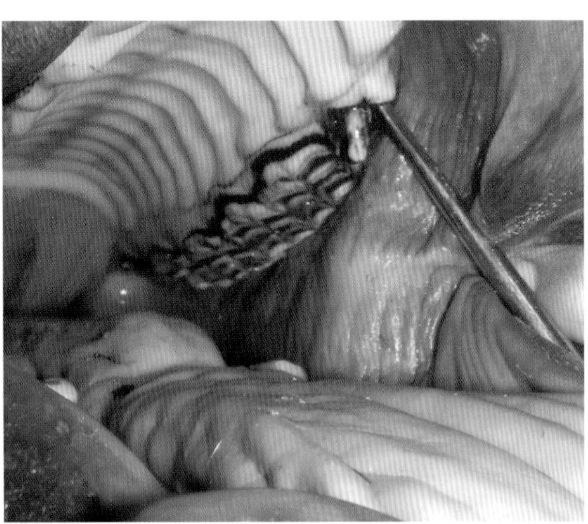

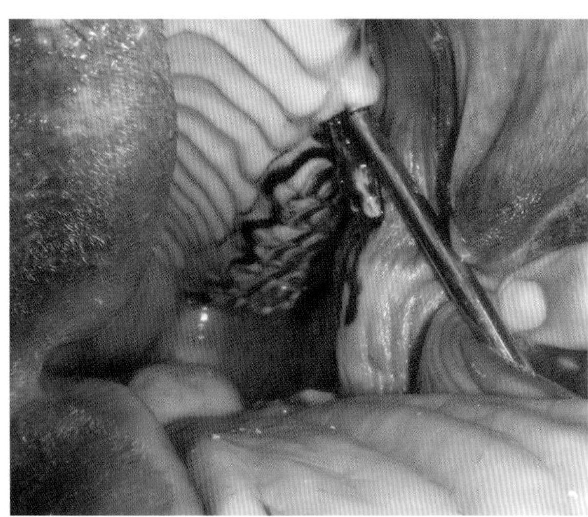

Top left and right: Extraction of a wolf tooth: a local anesthetic injection round the wolf tooth ensures that both the horse and the dental technician are at ease (left). The surrounding gum is loosened with a root extractor; the tooth is gradually worked loose (right).

Below left and right: In the ideal situation, the wolf tooth is lifted from the socket in this way (left and right pictures). After extraction, there will be a small opening in the gum. In order to allow the wound to heal undisturbed it is advised not to put a bit in the horse's mouth for about a week.

ministered, the wolf teeth, in most cases, can be calmly extracted. The gums surrounding the wolf tooth are loosened with a root lifter. Then, with a gradual application of pressure along the root, the fibers between the wolf tooth and the socket are severed. Often, it is even possible to finally lever the tooth out of its socket: if the wolf tooth is completely loosened, it can also be extracted with a pair of small forceps.

Even so, sometimes a wolf tooth breaks off with this technique. When the root has been broken off and is still too long, a root lifter can also be used to remove the rest of the root.

The sizes of wolf teeth are extremely variable: they are mostly about 1½ cm. Some are smaller than 1 cm; some can be as long as 4 cm. The size of the visible crown gives little indication of the length of the root. If the wolf tooth is already clearly moveable, this usually means that the root is partially broken up by pressure from the first permanent molar. If this wolf tooth is extracted, there is usually only a stump of root present.

Blind wolf teeth are removed in the same way as normal wolf teeth. These are usually oval-shaped with no clear root present.

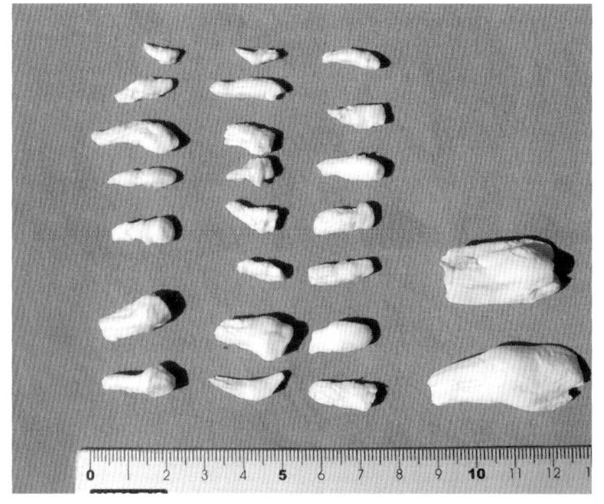

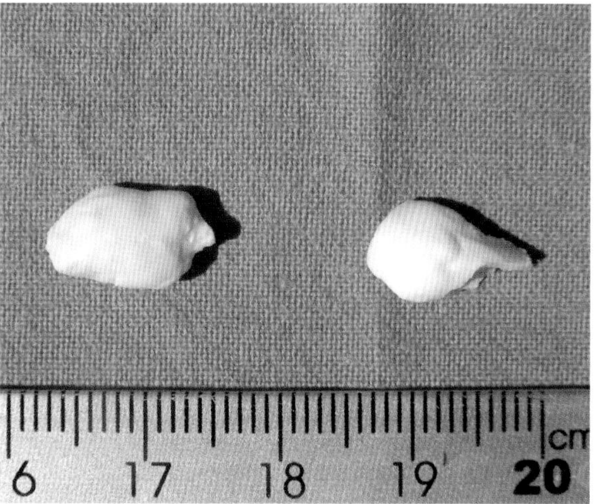

Left:
The size of wolf teeth is extremely variable. Most wolf teeth are about 1½ cm long and have a defined root. Some wolf teeth can be as long as 4 cm.

Right:
Blind wolf teeth are usually smaller than normal wolf teeth and frequently do not have a defined root.

Correction of Major Dental Defects

Major dental defects are always the result of abnormal abrasion. The principle of treatment for these defects is always the same: the taller parts are reduced so that a better sideways and forward and backward movement of the upper jaw in relation to the lower jaw is made possible. The accelerated abrasion of the molar opposite is then arrested, which means that in the future this tooth can regain its original form. If small corrections are carried out in a yearly dental examination, these defects are no longer seen.

The Molars

Hooks and ramps

Hooks usually develop on the front of the first upper molars and at the back of the last lower molars. Very often, they appear symmetrically placed on both sides of the set of teeth. The hooks are filed back to the normal height of the molar tables. Due to their position in the mouth, the hooks on the first molars are quite easy to reduce. The hooks on the last molars at the lower back are more difficult to reduce because of limited access to the back of the mouth. For these particular defects, the use of a power float is practically indispensable.

Sometimes the extra height is not limited to just the back or front of the molar table: the table of the first or last molar has a gradual slant of the whole surface, which ends in a hook. With these ramp teeth, the whole table is reduced to the normal table level. The opposite tooth is then no longer touching and, due to lack of abrasion, this tooth can gradually resume a normal visible crown height.

Step mouth

In a step mouth, the table of one molar is clearly taller than the neighboring teeth. This is sometimes caused by the loss of a molar in the opposite arcade of teeth. Due to the absence of abrasion the opposite tooth

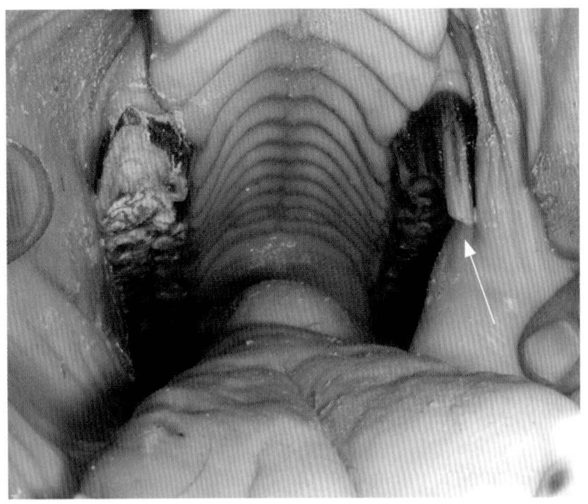

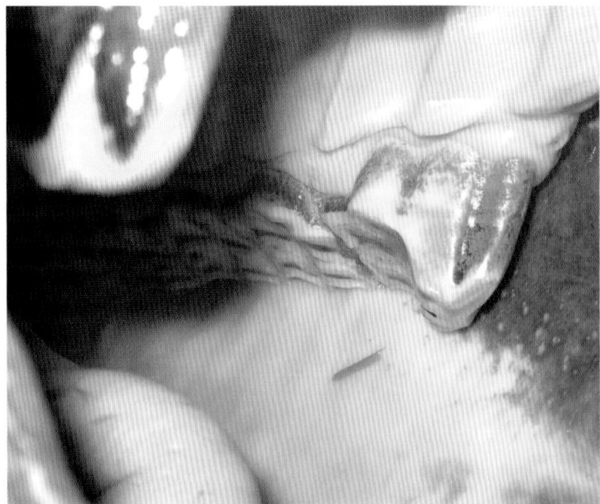

Left:
This horse had hooks on the front of both of the first upper molars; the hooks were 2 cm long. The hook on the left side has already been reduced. Notice the enormous difference in length between the fronts of both first upper molars.

Right:
According to the owner of this horse, the front hook had been treated six months before. Actually, only the front of the hook had been rounded off a little. This hook should really be reduced to the level of the table of the second molar.

becomes longer and longer. If this is corrected on an annual basis, the treatment is quite easy: but some horse owners do not realize the benefits to be had from a yearly dental inspection. Sometimes, the taller molar is 2 cm long and the correction must take place over several sessions. When too much crown is removed in one treatment, there is a chance that the root canal is opened and, in the long term, the tooth will be lost.

Wave mouth

A wave mouth has an upward or downward curve between the tables of the molars.

In this defect, several teeth are involved. Usually, the upward curve is on the lower arcade and involves the third and fourth molar; sometimes the second and fifth molars are also included in the curve. If it only concerns two molars (.08 and .09) then a correction in one treatment session is possible. When there are actually four molars involved, more sessions are needed otherwise the four molars (.07 to .10) would no longer be touching the opposite teeth and 70 percent of the tables in the whole molar arcade would no longer be operational. Moreover, the full pressure of grinding would then fall upon the first and last molars.

Shear mouth

In a shear mouth the angle of the tables is much too oblique. If this were to be corrected in one treatment session by reducing the long sides of the tables of the molars until a normal angle of 10 to 15 degrees was achieved, there would no longer be any surface contact possible over the whole length of the molar arcade. Therefore, this defect must often also be treated in several sessions. The cause of the shear mouth is also looked at and treated. In some horses, the situation is so serious that a full recovery is no longer possible. These horses must then be helped by being given a suitable diet.

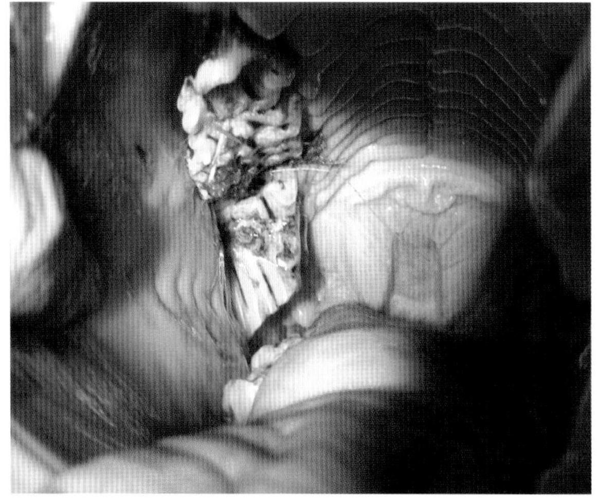

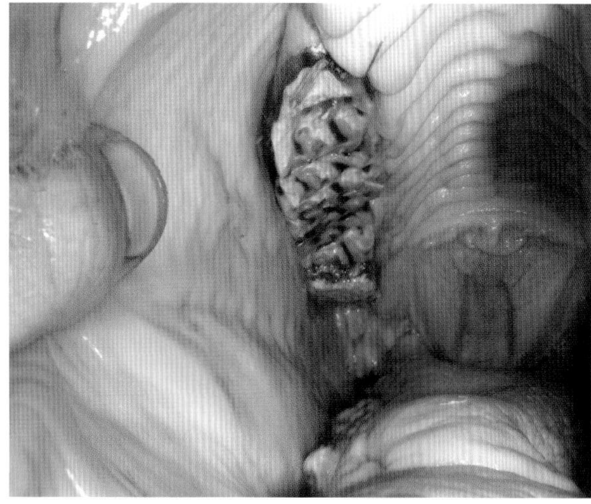

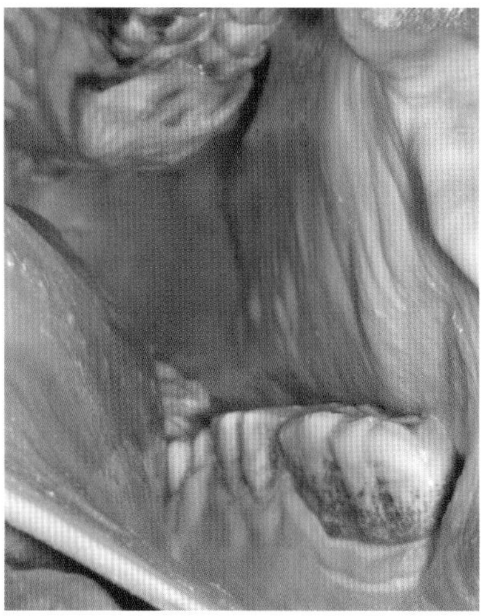

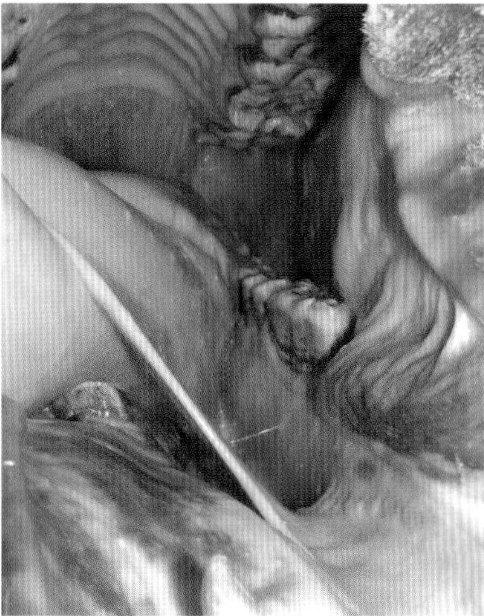

Top left and right:
A step tooth (110) in a 28-year-old pony that had serious chewing problems (squirreling of food in the mouth). This molar was 4 cm too long and had already caused a hole in the lower jaw. The tooth was cut back with a big pair of molar cutters and afterward trimmed and filed smooth (right). A day later, the pony could chew normally again. This pony should have been treated 10 years earlier!

Below left and right:
Left: A descending wave can be seen on the lower arcade of molars of this five-year-old. You can see that the upper molars have been reduced in height to allow for the possibility of the lower molars to grow up to a normal table level. Right: The same mouth one year after the former treatment. The descending wave has nearly disappeared. In the upper arcade, only the back of the fourth molar has to be reduced a little.

Diastema

Diastemas are small gaps between the molars that trap food. A diastema can be the cause of much pain as rough stalks of roughage can be caught between two neighboring teeth and press down on the gums. This causes periodontitis to form round the tooth concerned. If the gap is very narrow or is narrower at the top than underneath, the horse cannot remove the food with its tongue.

Often, other dental defects lead to the development of diastemas. The restoration of a good grinding surface thus forms the basis of the treatment. The diastemas are widened with suitable drills to create a space of about 6 mm between the molars so that the horse can remove any trapped food with its tongue. When the gums are badly affected, after a thorough cleaning, a plastic plug is placed between the molars for temporary protection. In this way the affected gums are protected and sometimes, this can result in a complete cure of the periodontitis. Other times, the horse is given an antibiotic treatment or an anti-inflammatory agent. After the treatment, the mouth is regularly rinsed with water. This is best done by holding the end of a garden hose in the horse's mouth for

Top two photos:
This horse had several diastemas. You can see the surrounding gums have been pushed down by several millimeters by the trapped roughage: this can be extremely painful. It's clear why the food could not be spontaneously removed by the horse: the opening at the table end is far narrower than the gum end.

Bottom six photos:
The first widening is made with a fine drill. Then by using larger and larger drill heads, the opening between the molars is widened to about 6 mm. Now, any food that becomes trapped in this opening can be easily removed by the horse itself.

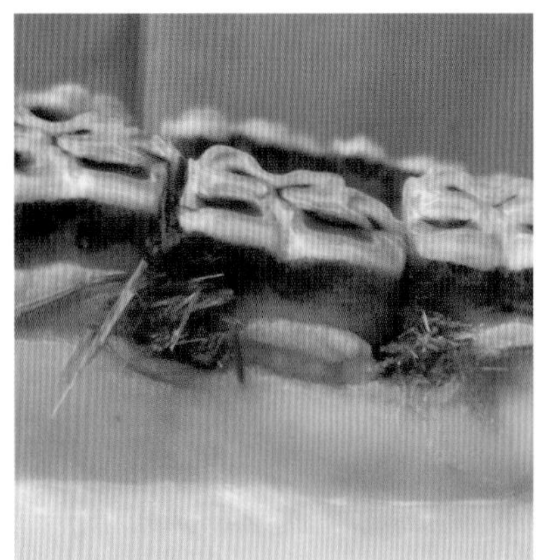

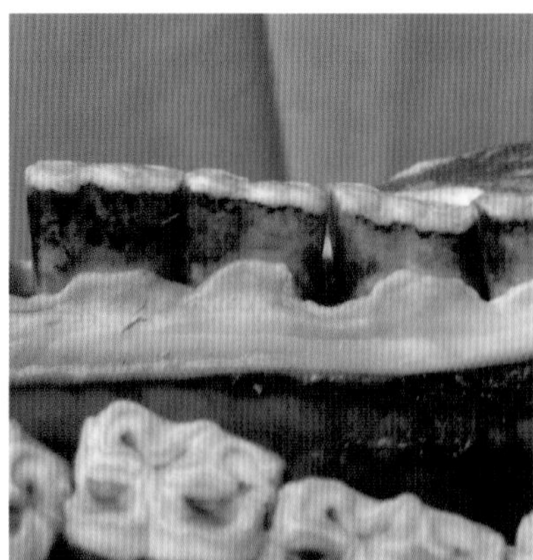

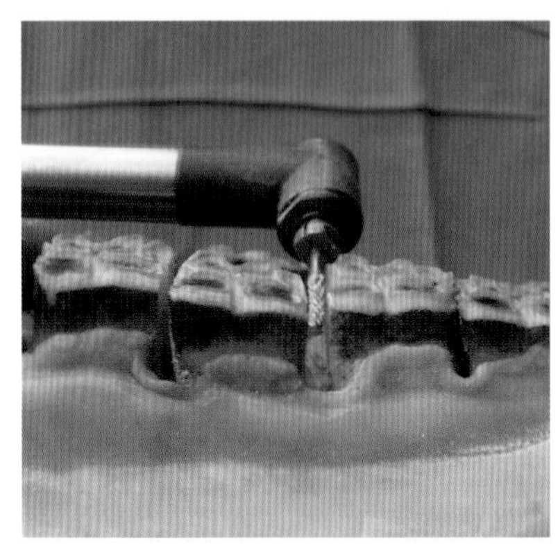

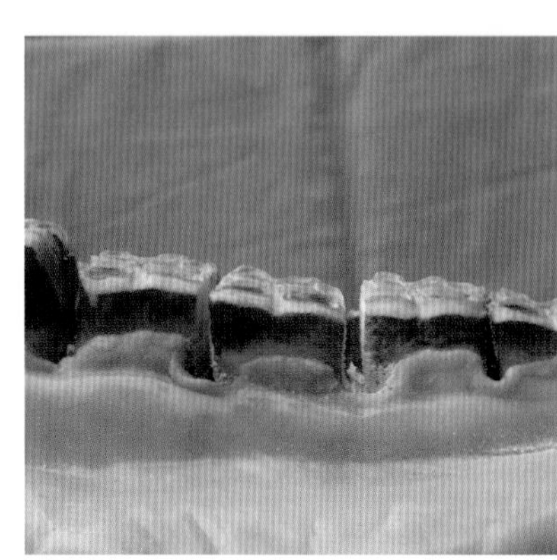

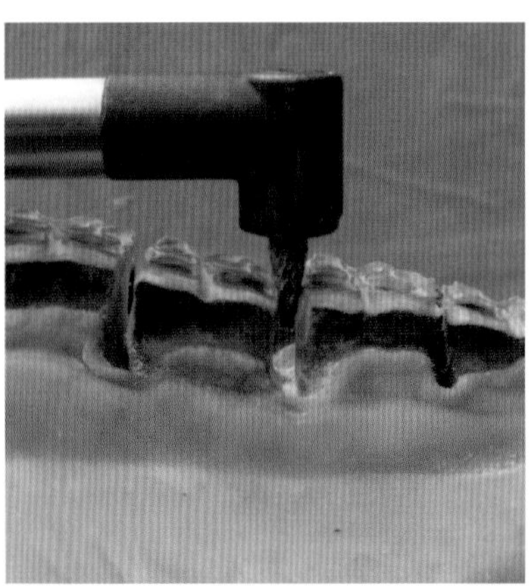

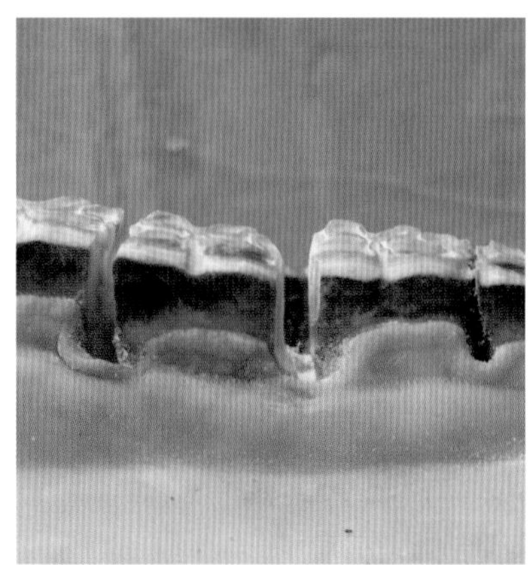

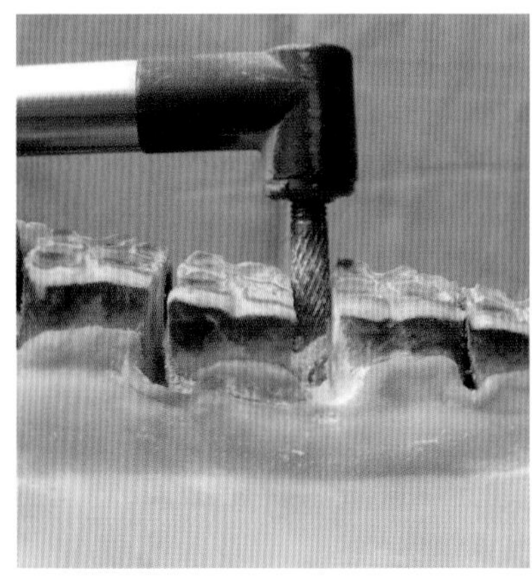

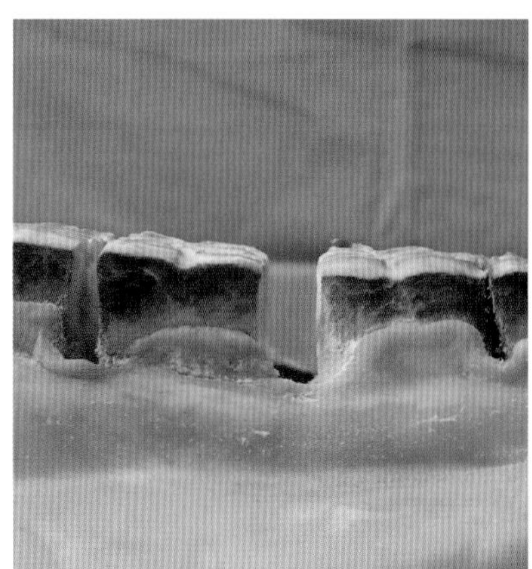

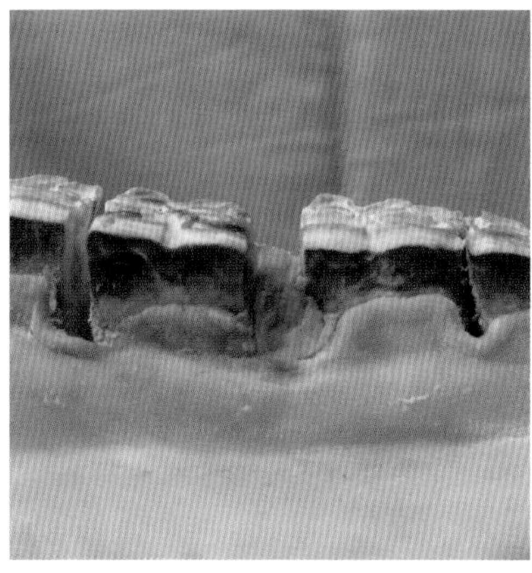

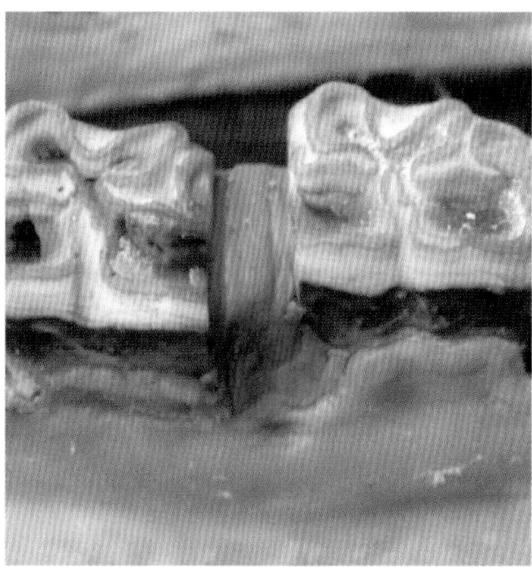

In order to protect the affected gums and give them the best chance of recovery, the gums are temporarily covered with a plastic plug.

the duration of about one minute.

In some cases, the periodontitis is so extensive that the molars have become loose, the socket has also been affected, and even food has entered via the root canal and into the sinus cavity. These horses then develop a suppurating sinusitis. It is obvious that for these advanced cases, there is sometimes no cure.

The Incisors

The incisors are treated only when the molars have been worked on. The taller parts of the incisors can be reduced with a hand or power float. Sometimes the incisors are reduced with thin diamond discs.

In order to have easy access to the incisors, a semi-hard, thick plastic tube is placed between the bars. This prevents the horse from bringing the incisors together and allows the tables to be floated.

Most horses find work on the incisors less pleasant than work on the molars. In such cases it is sometimes necessary to administer a local anesthetic.

In most incisor defects it is usually only necessary to reduce one or two incisors (step, ventral curvature, dorsal curvature or offset incisors). When there is an overbite or an underbite—where the nipping surface of the upper and lower jaws do not meet—all the incisors may be cut back.

Here too, the restriction applies of not removing too much of the crown in one session because the incisor root canal can be opened. This may lead to an infection of the root canal accompanied by the possible loss of the tooth as a result. Thus, several sessions are sometimes necessary to complete a full correction.

Extraction of an incisor or molar

There are several reasons for removing a horse's tooth:

- Loose teeth in an older horse
- A break in the vertical length of the tooth, usually preceded by caries and, in general, found in teeth of the upper jaw
- A break in a tooth from an outside trauma such as a kick from another horse

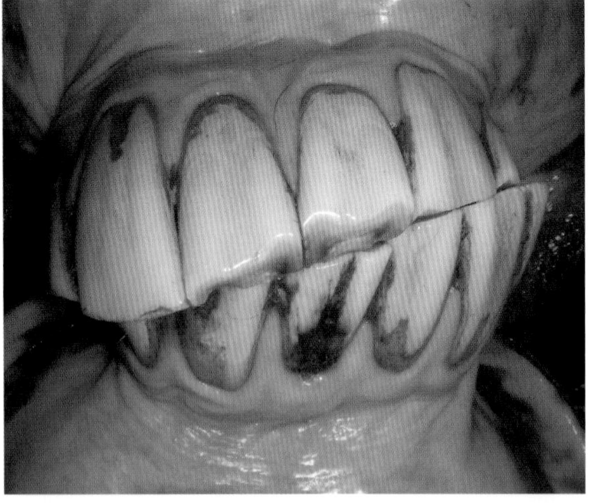

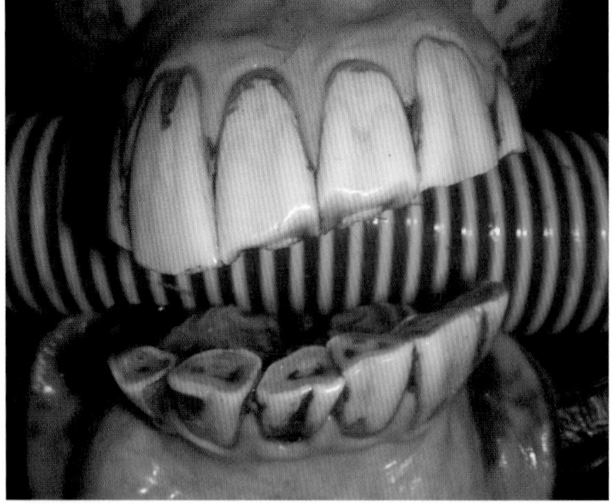

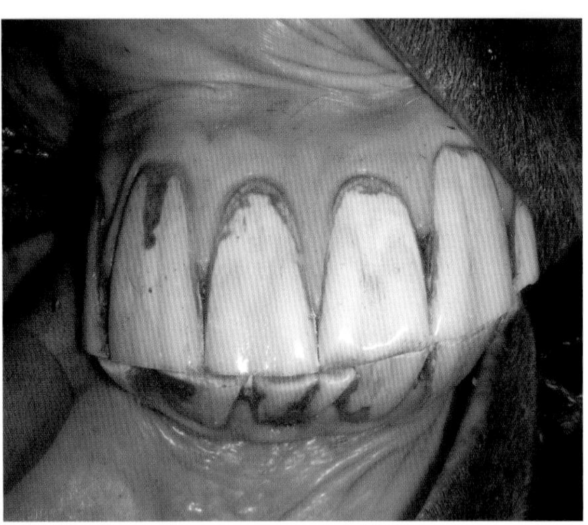

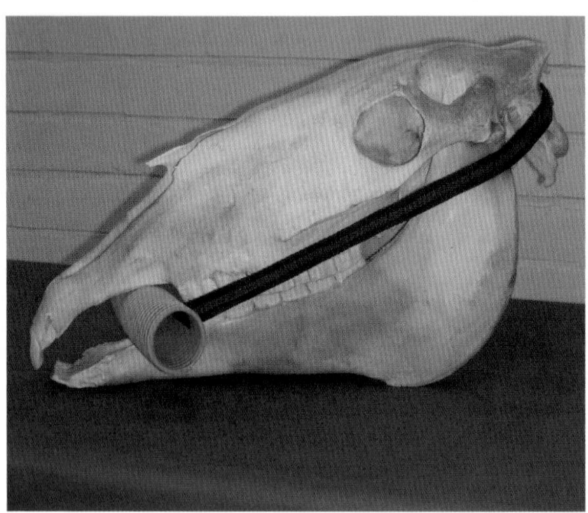

Top left:
Offset incisors

Top right:
With this mouth opened, notice that the right side of the upper incisors is shorter than the left side. The opposite is true of the lower incisors.

Below left:
The longer incisors have been floated, so we can say we have a satisfactory result after one session.

Below right:
An example of a semi-rigid plastic pipe that can be placed between the horse's bars. In this way, the incisors are held apart and easily treated.

- Advanced periodontitis
- Bacterial infection of the dental root accompanied or not by a suppurating fistulous opening on the outside of the head
- Bacterial infection of the dental root of one of the last four upper molars whereby the infection has spread through to the sinuses

Molars were already being extracted via the mouth from horses in a standing position in the nineteenth century. Considering that this was done without any kind of anesthetic, it was an extremely difficult task. With the introduction of better anesthetics in the second half of the last century, this method was replaced by surgical removal of molars under general anesthetic: the so-called "punching out" of the molars. With this, an opening was made through the bone on the outside of the horse's head above the molar concerned ("trephining"). Then a trephine punch was placed on the root of the molar and the molar was tapped with a hammer until it fell into the mouth. This technique for extracting molars was used everywhere until the end of the last century.

The number of complications and necessary second operations are really rather high with this technique. It is for this reason that in the

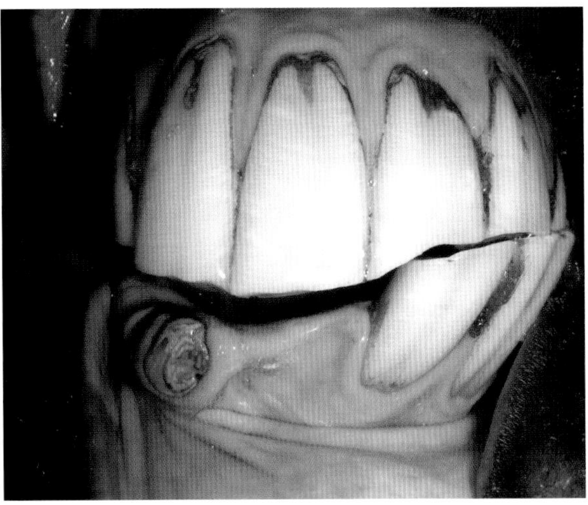

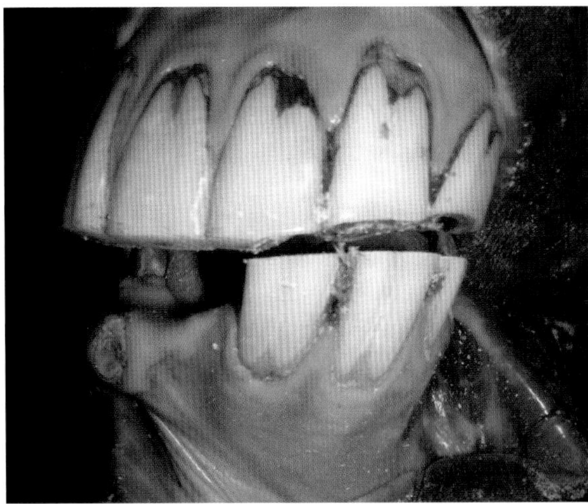

Top left:
Opposing incisors have grown down into the gap presented by missing teeth.

Top right:
In this picture, the correction is nearly complete: just another 2 mm shorter and the incisors can once again slide sideways across each other.

last 25 years a new surgical technique for the extraction of the first three molars—in both the upper and the lower jaw—has been employed. The mouth is reached via an incision in the cheek. The bony socket on the outside of the molar is removed. The molar is then extracted sideways from the socket and the incision in the cheek is stitched up. There are fewer complications in the application of this technique.

However, in recent years there has been a return to the oldest method of all: the extraction of molars via the mouth. These days, however, modern anesthetics and local anesthetic techniques are used so that the treatment can be carried out in a humane manner. The chance of complication is also much smaller; the technique can often be used on standing horses; the follow-up treatment and the process of recovery are much quicker. Above all, this method is usually much, much cheaper. If a complete

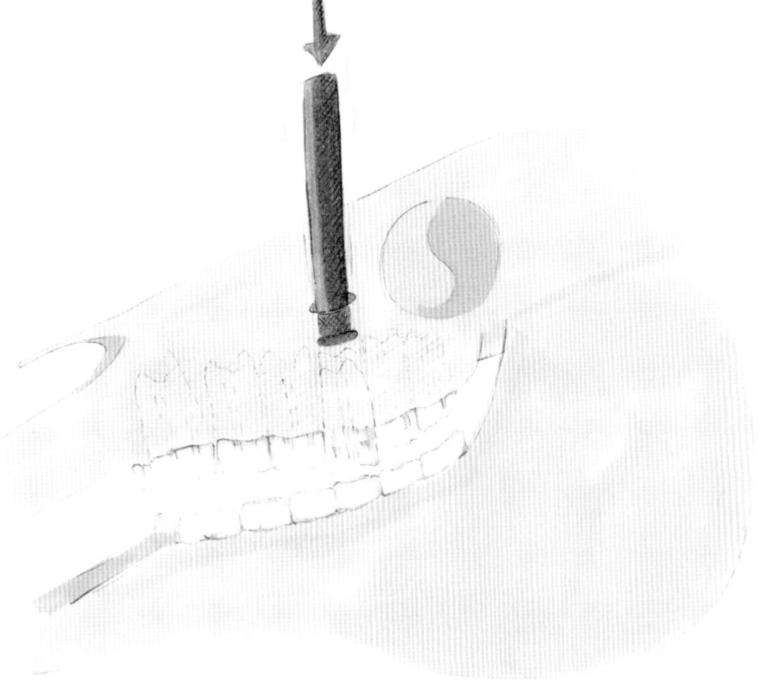

When "punching out" a molar, an opening is made on the outside of the head. The molar is knocked out into the mouth with a hammer and trephine punch.

This horse had the third upper molar removed via a crescent-shaped incision in its cheek.

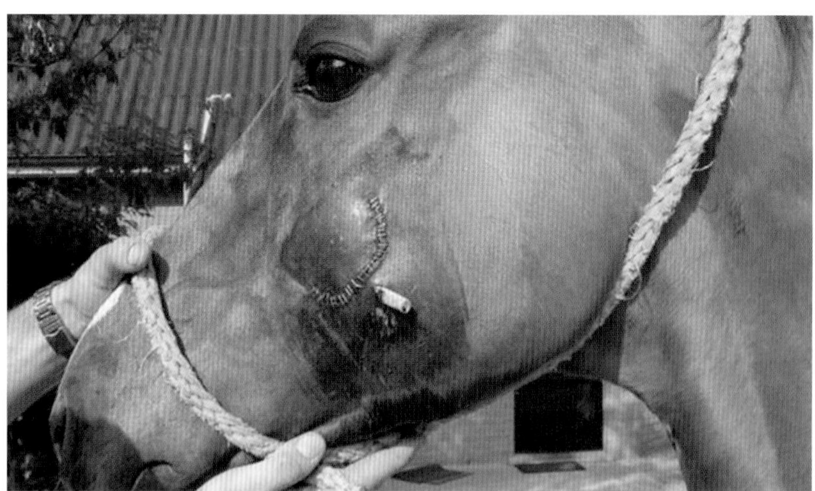

extraction does not succeed by this method, then you can always resort to the surgical removal of the rest of the remaining tooth.

With the use of sedatives, common painkillers and local anesthetic techniques, extraction can take place via the mouth in a standing horse. This method is unsuccessful with some horses because of their temperament; in such cases the same technique is applied but under general anaesthetic.

When extracting via the mouth, first the gums round the tooth concerned are loosened. In order to pull loose the fibers that hold the molar in the socket, a wedge-shaped pair of pliers—the molar spreader—is clamped to the front and back of the tooth concerned between the other molars. The wedge shape of the molar spreader commences to force the tooth away from the neighboring molars. Then, the visible crown of the tooth is firmly clamped with a pair of forceps for molar extraction. By a slow horizontal movement with the end of the forceps, we endeavor to loosen the tooth round its longitudinal axis. When it is clear that the tooth is moving, we often hear a squishing sound; frothy blood also arises up round the tooth from the socket. In young horses, it can take at least

Below left:
A split molar can often be extracted via the mouth while the horse is standing because the fragments are only attached on one side to the surrounding tissue.

Below right:
This picture shows the two fully extracted fragments.

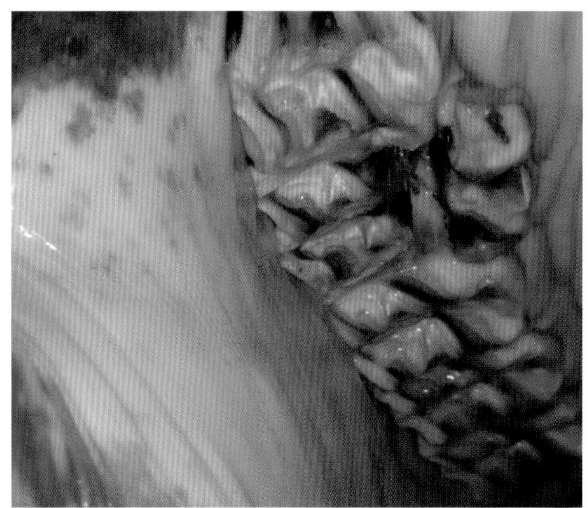

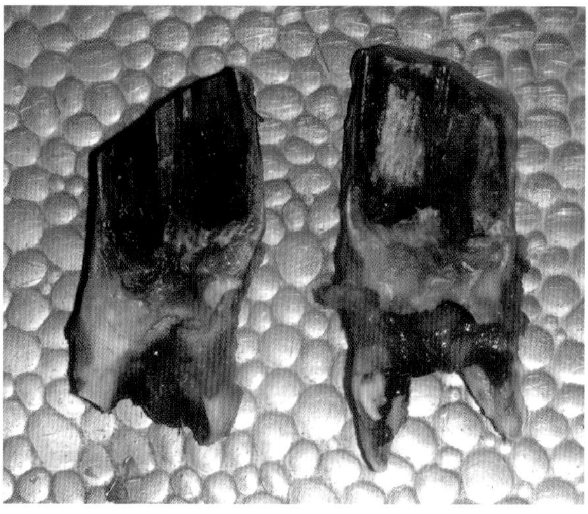

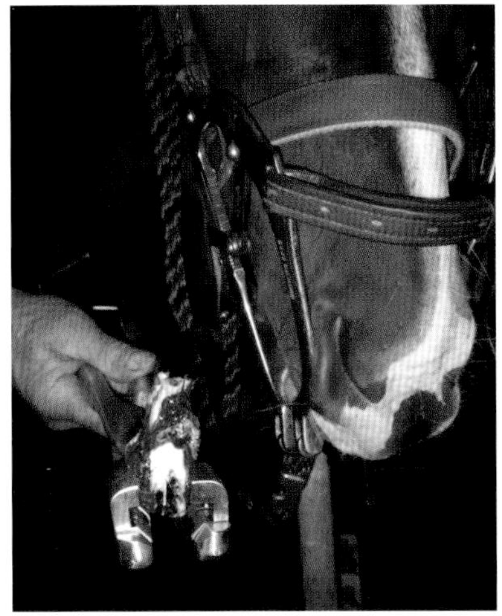

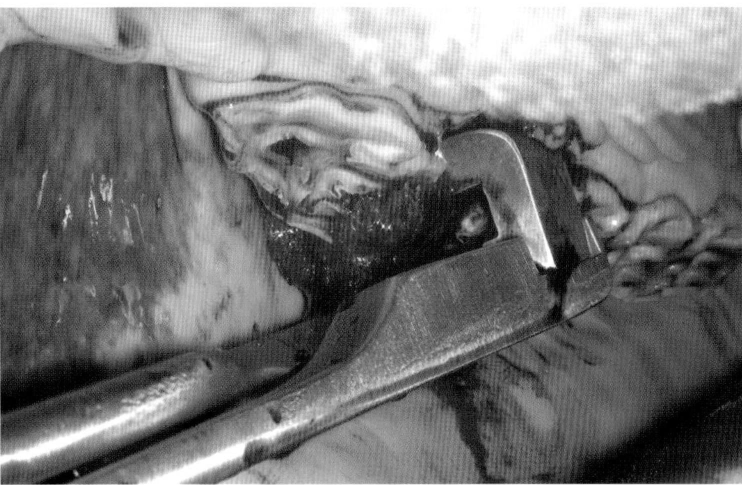

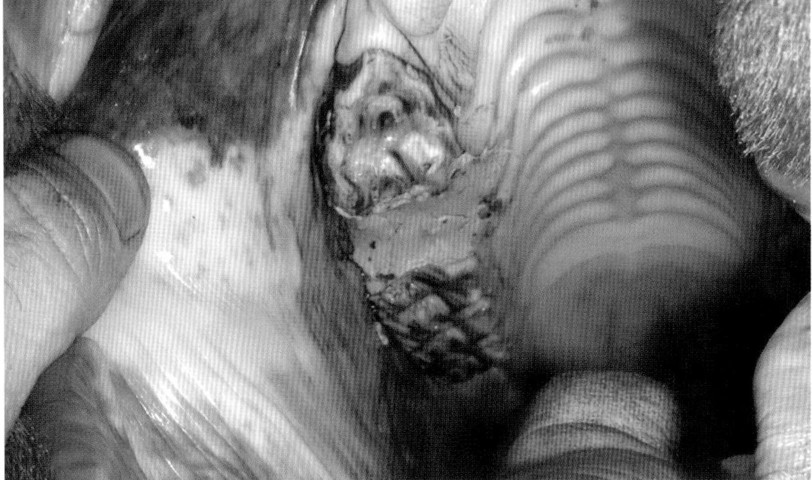

Top left:
This complete molar was removed via the mouth of a standing horse. Sometimes, achieving this result can take two hours of careful prising.

Top right:
This picture shows a molar extraction in a standing horse. The molar is gradually worked loose with molar forceps. As soon as a squishing sound is heard and frothy blood arises round the tooth, the tooth is loose enough to begin pulling out the tooth.

Below:
After the tooth has been extracted, the resulting gap in the socket is filled with a plastic plug to prevent food accumulating there. When the hollow becomes filled with tissue, the plug can be removed after two or three weeks. Horses frequently lose the plug before then, however.

a couple of hours before the tooth is loose enough to start pulling. Using stronger and broader sideways movements of the forceps in order to hasten this process often leads to a fracture of the tooth concerned and will put an end to extraction via the mouth. When the tooth is loose enough, a fulcrum is placed between the teeth in front and the handles of the forceps. By pressure on the handles of the forceps—outside the mouth—the molar is then levered out of the socket.

This technique is always applied to older horses that have loose teeth. The reserve crown and the root in these animals are relatively short due to advanced abrasion. Sometimes the teeth of old horses are so loose that they can be pulled out with the fingers.

When there is a lengthwise fracture in the root, the two halves of the tooth have often been pushed apart by the chewing of food and consequently each half is fixed to the socket on only one side. Due to this, the two halves can often be extracted via the mouth.

In young horses, the socket is still rather deep so is filled with a rubber-like plug after the tooth is extracted. In this way, no food can become wedged in the hole; the plug is removed after two or three weeks.

The healthy molar on the right of this picture has sharply defined roots. At left, the roots of a loose molar that was extracted. Note the knob-like cementum deposits on the roots of this tooth.

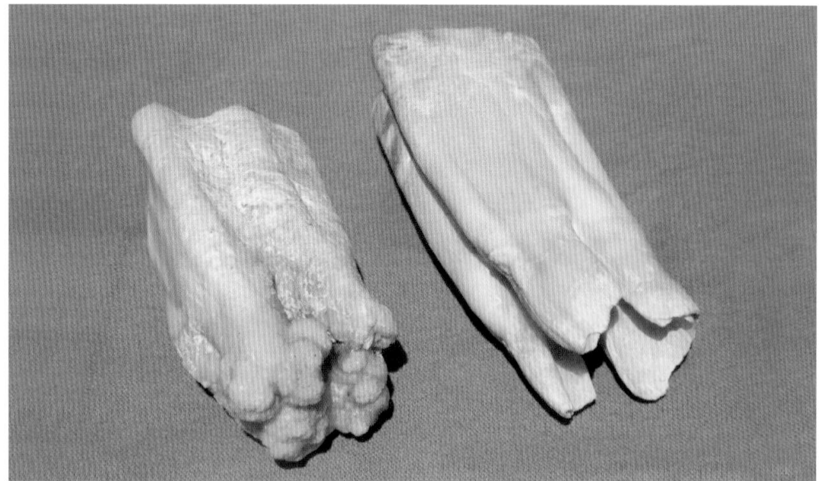

When there is an infected root in one of the four last upper molars, the sinus cavity is often filled with pus. In these circumstances, the choice is usually to "punch out" the molar under general anesthesia. At the same time, the sinus cavity can be cleaned and rinsed out. The surgical punching out of molars and the treatment of the accompanying sinus infection is only carried out in specialist equine clinics.

The ideal treatment of a bacterial root infection of a molar is actually by root canal treatment. At the height of the affected molar root, the bone along the outside is removed. The affected molar root is then cleaned out and filled with a special substance. In this way, the tooth can remain in the mouth and no additional defects can arise such as an opposite molar becoming higher by growing into the ensuing opening of an extracted tooth. Only dental root infections that answer to very specific criteria can be considered for this treatment. Otherwise, this method of treatment is seldom successful for completely removing the infection; often we nevertheless must resort to the full extraction of a tooth.

CHAPTER 16

The Importance of a Properly Fitted Bit

Although bits are not part of dental care, I am, however, confronted nearly every day with the results of a poorly fitting bit or incorrect use of the reins. Therefore, I would like to offer a few comments about the bit.

The bit serves to provide subtle communication with the head of the horse. Sometimes, however, I see the bit being used to stabilize a rider and keep him sitting upright in the saddle. An independent seat is the first requirement for correct contact with the bit. I often hear talk about "subtle use of the reins" but a bad seat results in bad hands: at every step, the hands move 5 cm up and down, or backward and forward. This is not a "subtle" use of the reins, and the horse's mouth can be damaged. Because the horse inevitably shows resistance, there is even less chance of subtlety, and a vicious circle is set up. The claim that a horse with a painful mouth reacts to rein aids more sensitively has no grounds whatsoever. Most horses have the tendency to fight pain if they can't escape it. These horses will then display even more resistance when more pressure is put on the mouth.

Pressure—and its release—is what a horse should be able to understand. When you apply pressure and your horse stops, you reward it by discontinuing the pressure after completion of the exercise. The majority of horses rapidly understand this. However, if the reins are continually

Left:
The sides of the tongue and the bars of the mouth of this driving horse have obviously been irritated by the action of the bit. Discomfort guaranteed!

Right:
This dressage horse's tongue has been damaged by the action of the curb bit. You can hardly expect a willing acceptance of the bit with injuries such as these in the mouth.

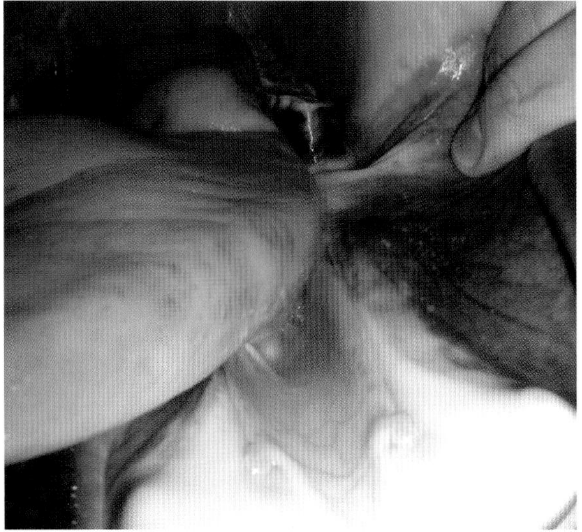

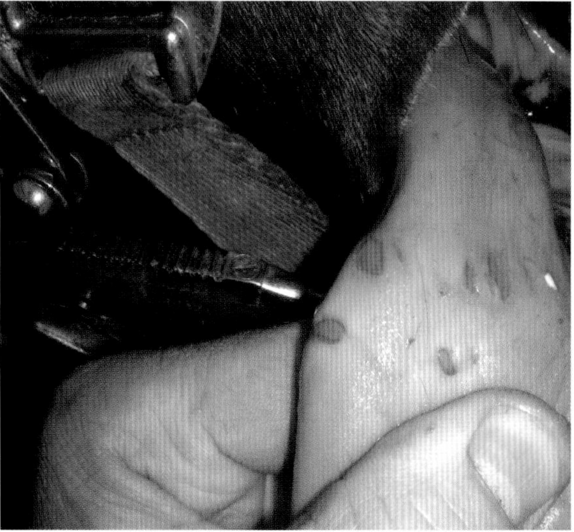

pulled and the pressure on the mouth isn't released, in the end, the horse reacts in a confused manner.

The bit is positioned in a very sensitive place in the mouth. A well-fitting bit lies over the tongue just in front of the first molars. In applying pressure with the reins, first the corners of the mouth are lightly moved then when more pressure is applied, it is received on the tongue and when there is even more pressure applied, it is possible to have the bit be felt on the bars. In fact, a well-schooled horse reacts to the first signal of the pressure to come. Even before you can apply stronger pressure in the mouth, the well-schooled horse has already reacted and further pressure is no longer required. In this type of riding, the rein aids are barely visible. The horse then happily accepts the bit because there is no more pulling in its mouth. I'm absolutely convinced that a horse that accepts the bit can be ridden with all kinds of bits. Though, frequently, all kinds of bits are tried in order to have the horse accept the bit—the world is thus upside down!

When the horse experiences pain somewhere in the mouth, this has a bad effect on its concentration during work. Just imagine if you had to concentrate when doing a job for your boss while you had a toothache. For example, cheek injuries may be seen in the horse's mouth because, by using a high noseband, the cheeks are pressed against the outer edge of the tables of the upper molars at this spot. If the horse hasn't had any preventive dental care, enamel points are pressed into the cheeks and cause lesser or greater injuries. When these horses open their mouths in order to evade the pain while being ridden, the rider often then tightens the noseband yet another notch in order make the horse keep its mouth closed. This results in even more pain from the enamel points pressing into the cheeks. If the rider loosens the noseband by a couple of notches instead, and notices that the horse seems to go better, he would know it would be a good idea to have the horse's mouth examined.

Some horses will try and relieve the pain in their mouths with their tongue. By repositioning their tongues in their mouths, the pressure from the bit can be born differently. Then the tongue is pushed forward outside the mouth or hung sideways outside the mouth—something that nobody likes to see. Even after correction of the defect that provoked it, it is often very difficult to break horses of this habit.

A bit should fit the horse well, and each horse should thus have its own bit. A bit should not be too wide: this can cause it to move back and forth in the mouth and with a jointed snaffle or French link (multi-jointed) snaffle, the contact will then be with the bars instead of the middle of the tongue. When a curb bit with a tongue port is too big, it can bang against the molars. When the bit is too narrow, there will be continuous pressure on the corners of the mouth and the cheeks from the rings; this will also cause pressure on the outside edge of the molars. I prefer to see the bit extending beyond the corners of the mouth by a half to one centimeter. You can determine the height of the bit in the

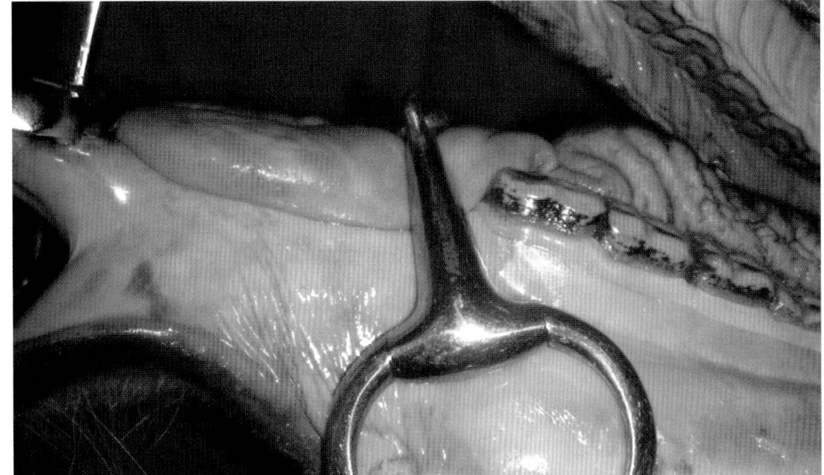

This is the normal position of the jointed snaffle. The bit lays a couple of centimeters in front of the first molars; it rests on the middle of the tongue and just touches the upper outer edges of the bars.

mouth by counting the number of creases in the corners of the mouth: there should be one or two with a bit that is hanging in the mouth in the correct position.

The thickness of the bit is determined by the intensity of effect desired on the mouth. The thinner the bit, the more severe the effect will be. On the other hand, the bit can also be too thick. Anatomical limitations have to be taken into consideration concerning the thickness of a bit but, in any case, it must lie comfortably in the mouth. In most Warmbloods, there is a space of 3 to 4 cm between the upper and lower jaw at the height of the bars but some horses only have a space of not more than 2 cm. In this case, if you put in a bit of 2 cm thick, the horse would have to keep its mouth open. The size of the tongue port in the curb bit should be considered from the same standpoint. A curb bit with 2 cm room for the tongue will certainly guarantee more freedom of movement for the tongue. However, if the space between the upper and lower jaw is really limited, the action of the lower shank (or cheek piece) rotates the curb bit upward in the mouth and the raising of the bit will then press into the horse's hard palate. The question is whether the advantage of more

Below left:
This is the position of the curb bit with a tongue port when there is no traction on the lower shanks.

Below right:
As soon as the reins are pulled, the curb bit rotates in the mouth; the tongue is then enclosed under the curb bit, which subsequently presses onto the sensitive upper side of the bars.

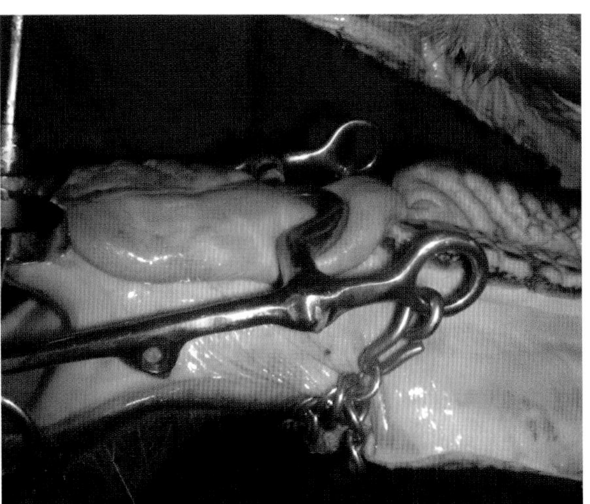

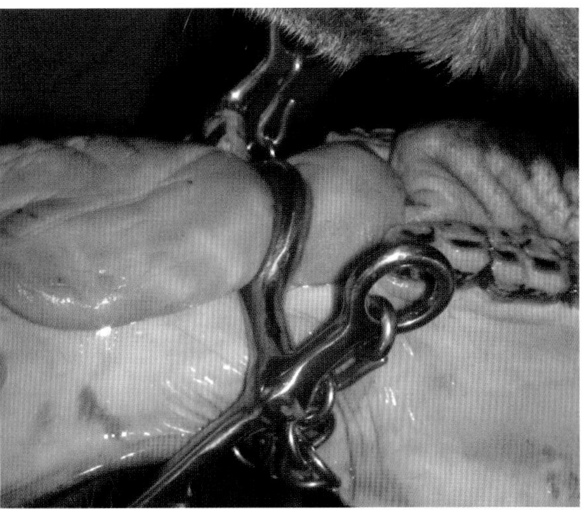

freedom of the tongue is worth the pain in the hard palate. A well-fitting bit should therefore be tried on your horse at home with careful consideration for the type of mouth it has.

I would also very much like to bring to your attention the difference between the pressure exercised by a snaffle and that of a curb bit with a curb chain.

Using a jointed snaffle or straight bar snaffle (this is a curb bit without a curb chain) the traction of the hands on the reins is transferred directly as pressure in the horse's mouth. With a jointed or French link snaffle, the pressure is more equally distributed over the tongue, the bars and the corners of the mouth than it is by a straight bar snaffle. With a straight bar snaffle, initially the pressure is felt on the tongue that is positioned higher than the bars. As more pressure is applied, the tongue is flattened on the bars and if the tongue is pulled away, the pressure comes directly onto the bars.

The Curb Bit

Riding with a curb bit and curb chain is another order of intensity entirely. Here, the intensity is not only determined by the pulling power of the reins but also by the leverage action of the lower shanks (or cheek pieces). This is determined by the distance to the center of the curb from the attachment to the reins as contrasted with the distance to the center of the curb from the attachment to the curb chain. If, for example, there is a ratio of 4:1 and there are 11 lbs (5 kilos) of traction power on the reins, this translates into 44 lbs (20 kilos) of pressure in the horse's mouth. Taking this over two hands, I am then talking about 88 lbs (40 kilos) of pressure in the horse's mouth when each hand has a traction power of 11 lbs (5 kilos).

The attachment of a curb chain is the deciding factor in this issue. When the curb chain is just left loose, then you have the same power ratio as you do with a jointed bit. When you have the curb chain very tight, even the slightest pressure from your hand will cause enormous pressure in the mouth of the horse. However, if you slightly loosen the curb chain, when you take up your reins lightly, there is a slight rotation of the curb bit in the mouth. In this way, the horse understands that the rotation of the curb is the warning signal before more pressure is exercised.

A well-schooled riding horse, with this signal in mind, has some indication of what is expected of it. In this way, rein aids can also be applied very finely. Therefore, with a fully trained horse and an experienced rider's hand, a curb bit and curb chain can produce a beautiful performance. However, if such a system is used because a horse does not go on the bit or it is used by an inexperienced rider it becomes a true instrument of torture.

To discover the effect of this pressure for yourself, try the following

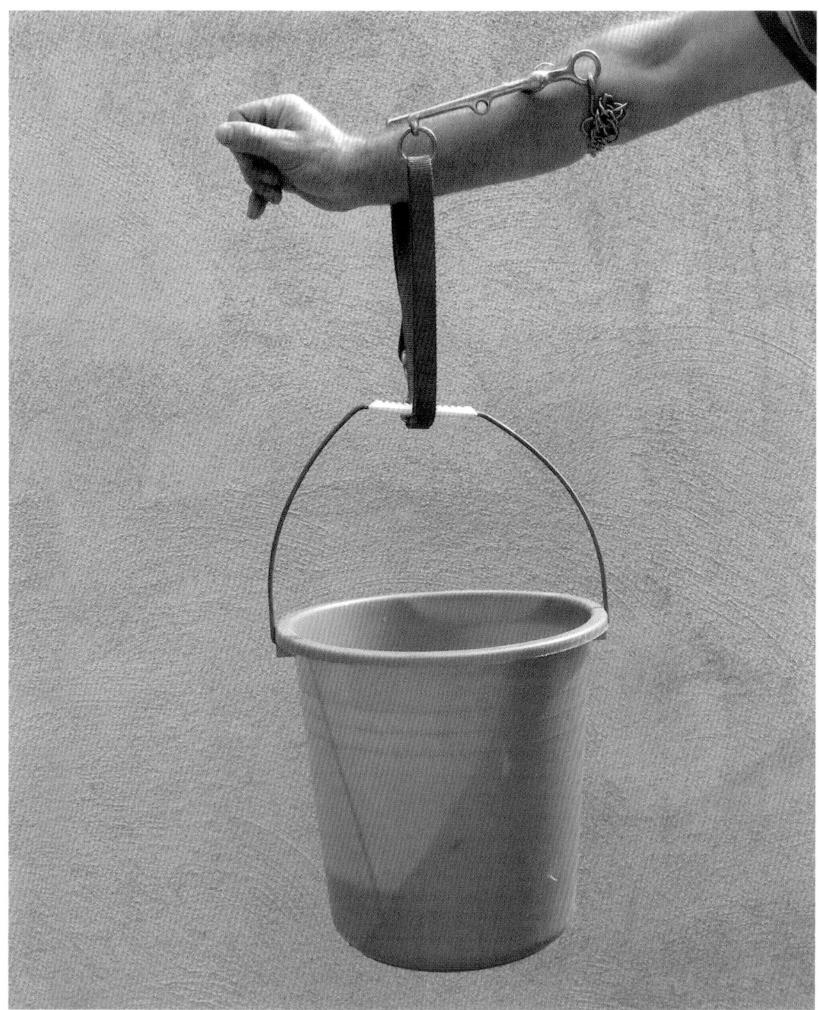

Everybody who works with a double bridle should first try this experiment. Hang a bucket with 1 to 2 gallons (5 to 10 liters) of water on your curb bit as illustrated in the picture. Then lift the bucket up for 10 seconds. Try this first without attaching the curb chain and afterwards, repeat the experiment with a tightly attached curb chain. This experiment will, without a doubt, lead you to a much more careful and sensitive use of the double bridle in the future.

experiment. Lay a jointed snaffle bit on top of your lower arm. Take a piece of rope and thread it through the handle of a bucket and attach both ends to the rings of the snaffle. Now put 1 to 2 gallons (5 to 10 liters) of water in the bucket. Lift the bucket from the ground with your lower arm and hold it for 10 seconds. Easily done! Now put the curb bit on your lower arm and fix the curb chain tightly underneath your lower arm. This still feels comfortable. Now, in the same way as before, put the rope through the handle of the bucket and attach the rope ends to the ends of the lower shanks of the curb. Lift up the bucket for 10 seconds, keeping your lower arm horizontal and see how this feels! Without a doubt you will now use the curb bit and curb chain with a great deal more respect for your horse.

CHAPTER 17

Dental Care for Miniature Horses

Dental defects are common to all breeds, though I see defects due to abnormal abrasion of the molars less frequently in ponies than in horses.

However, in comparison to other breeds, I see more dental problems in miniature horses. Indeed, the breeder's goal is to produce the smallest horse possible with as fine a head as possible. However, it has been proven in genetic studies that the teeth reduce in size far less quickly than the jaw that holds them. Thus, a miniature horse's teeth are not much smaller than the teeth of a horse weighing 1000 lbs. Frequently, we also see that some molars are implanted outside the normal arcade of teeth: this causes abnormal abrasion in the opposite molars.

Other dental defects caused by abnormal abrasion of the molars are also common, such as the formation of hooks and a wave mouth. We often see an overbite or an underbite in the incisors. Sometimes the space in the lower jaw or the upper jaw is too narrow for the permanent incisors and these are then implanted in a twisted way. These miniatures are usually brought to us rather late in the day for dental examination and treatment.

The space in the mouth where the treatment must take place is also rather cramped. It is often necessary to use suitably small instruments.

Left:
Miniature horses often display dental defects. The mouth is, as it were, too small to hold so many large teeth. These animals can be properly treated with instruments of a suitable size.

Right:
The lower jaw of this Miniature is not big enough for all its incisors. Incisor 302 has turned 90 degrees due to lack of space.

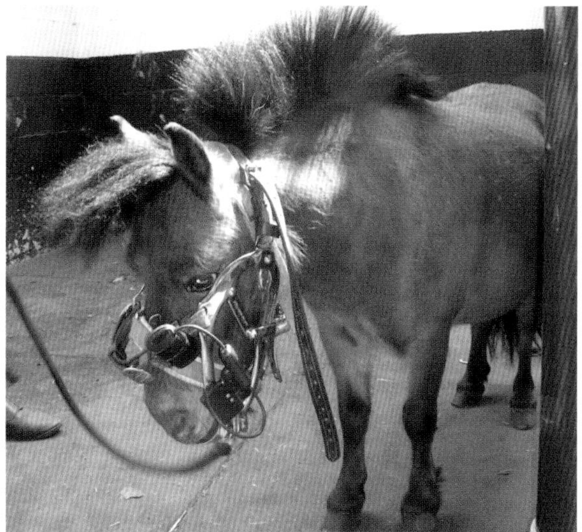

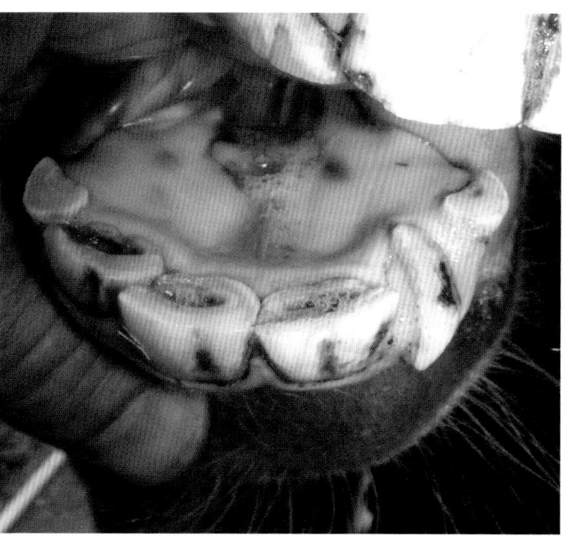

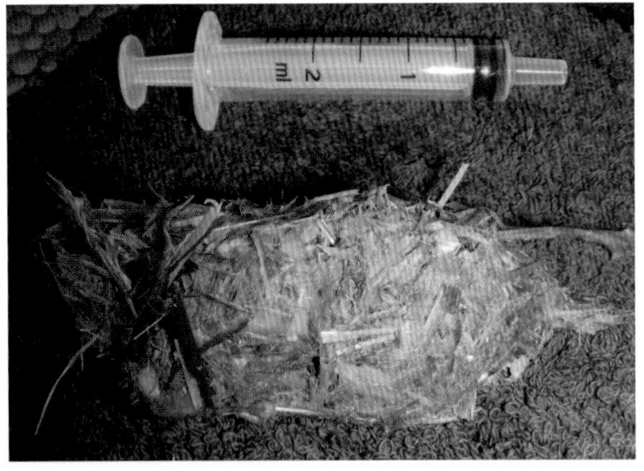

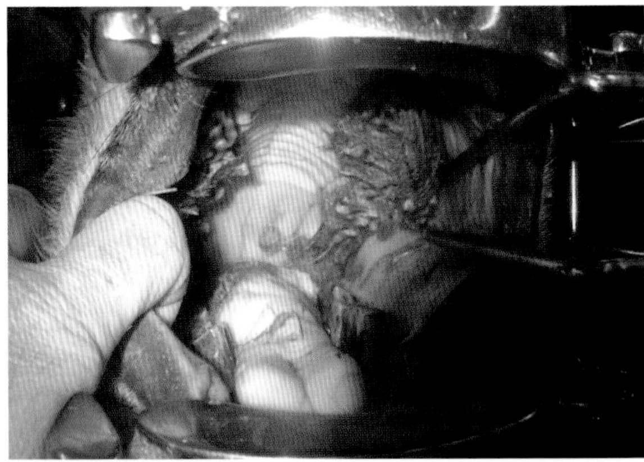

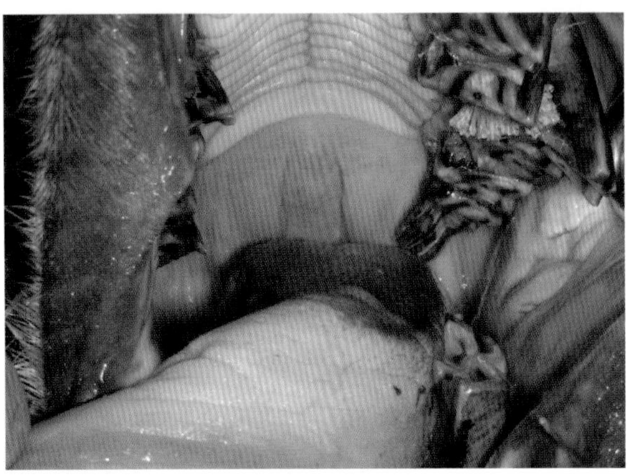

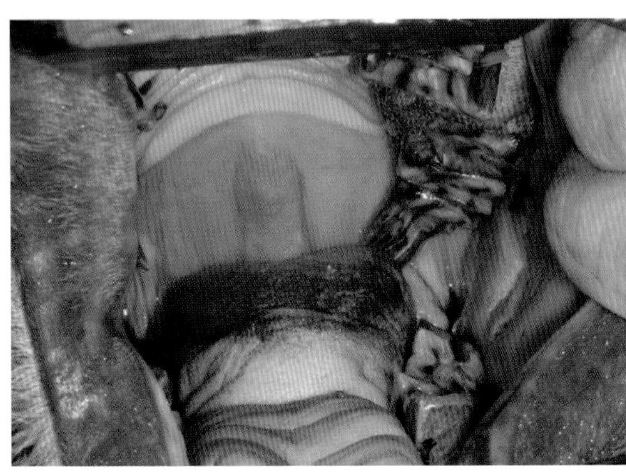

Top left:
Compacted food that a Miniature donkey had been squirreling in its mouth inside both cheeks; it had been doing this for more than a year.

Top right:
When the mouth was opened, the grass collected on the outside and round the back of the molars was easy to see.

Below left:
After the mouth was rinsed, the reason for squirreling food became clear: the third molar was slightly loose and was pressing into the cheek. There was a large hook on the last upper molar that was touching the tongue.

Below right:
The abnormal molars were extracted from both sides (108 and 208). Subsequently, the large hook was cut back. A few days after treatment, the donkey was back to eating normally.

Most of these horses are kept as pets and the characteristic of being "well behaved" among them has quite a different meaning from what we would call well behaved in a saddle horse. Therefore, sedation is usually required when treating these animals even when using hand floats only.

CHAPTER 18

Dental Care for Older Horses

From the age of twenty, horses are considered "older." If horses are enjoying their old age, they can quite well live to 30 or 40 years old. However, the teeth continue erupting further and further from their sockets and, thus, the reserve crown becomes shorter and shorter within the socket.

The last part of the reserve crown and root of the molar contain no enamel. This means that the structure is far less hard. From the moment that these parts are used for chewing, the rest of the tooth will wear down very quickly. From this time, we call them "soft" molars. In the end, the roots of the molars gradually fall out.

Research has show that 60 percent of horses older than 15 years have abnormal abrasion of the molars and periodontitis is present. Due to the development of abnormal pressure on the molars and the loosening of the tissues round the tooth, the loss of the molars is even more accelerated.

In these horses, there is often a lot of plaque present round the canines, the corner incisor (.03) and on the outside of the first upper molars. This can lead to the development of gingivitis around the tooth. Of course, the plaque can be removed but it returns within a month in some horses.

Dental defects in the older horse often give rise to problems because the horse cannot take in enough food and cannot grind it finely enough. These horses also produce less saliva. Indeed, saliva flows during chewing. This process allows the food taken in to be digested and to descend into the intestinal tract. Frequently, long fibers of hay or whole grains of corn can be seen in the droppings. Due to insufficient grinding, the

Left and right:
The upper molars of a 28-year-old horse. The fourth upper molar (209) is missing so the opposite molar (309) has subsequently grown up into the opening; the adjacent tooth (210) has moved forward.

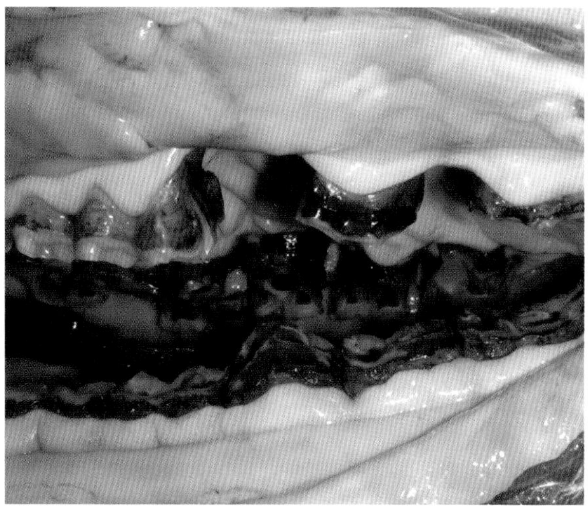

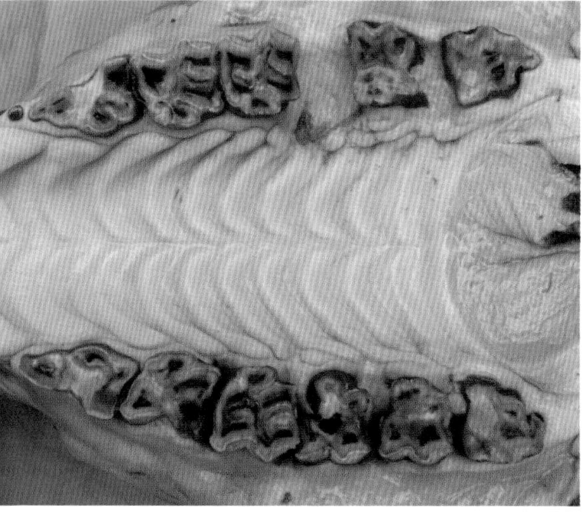

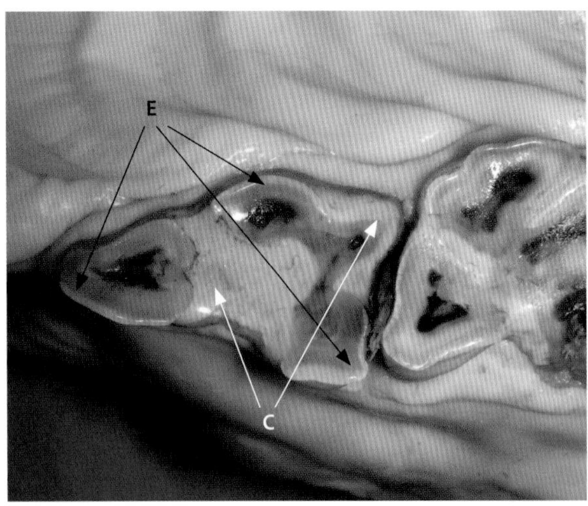

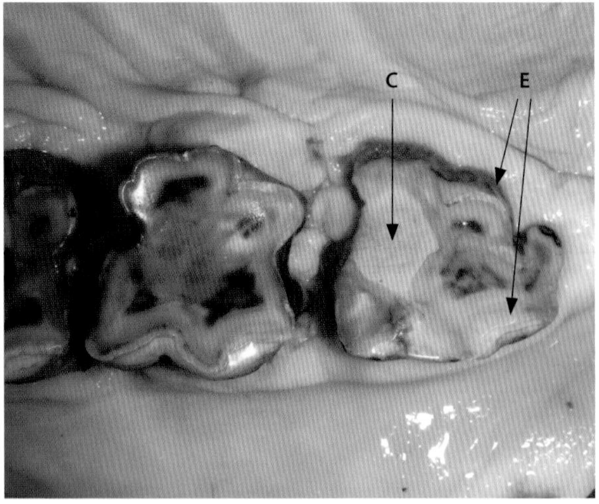

Left and right:
On the first molar (left) and the last molar (right) you can see that the hard enamel (E) has nearly completely disappeared and mostly cementum (C) remains. This is what we call "soft" molars. These will wear down much more quickly because they are less hard.

starch present in the grains of corn is not exposed to the digestive process by the body's own enzymes in the stomach and the small intestines. A stream of too much undigested starch to the appendix and to the large intestine can lead to an imbalance of the micro-flora present. This can result in problems such as colic or watery droppings. When roughage is not sufficiently ground up into smaller parts, the contact surface of these nutrients is not adequate enough to make good bacterial digestion possible. Thus, the horse takes in enough nutrients but is not able to benefit from them to the full.

If an older horse is no longer able to chew and grind normal rations (grass, hay and grains) then other measures must be taken in order to give it sufficient energy-supplying nutrients. When there are dental problems, older horses can more easily take in short grass than long and hard hay. When horses are put out to grass, older horses often grow fatter but they lose weight again when brought back. When no grass is available, it can be replaced by chopped hay or by alfalfa (Lucerne) pellets.

Concentrates in the form of horse pellets are easier to grind finely than whole grains so are therefore an advantage for older horses. What is more, during the production process of concentrates, they can also be briefly heated (extruded or expanded); this allows the starch to be partly released so the horse can utilize it more easily. Do not, however, give your older horse unlimited concentrates or commercial mash. This will result in the intake of too many sugars and starch that can cause digestive difficulties.

Significantly more energy can be taken in with the same amount of food by augmenting the amount of fat in the rations. One can do this by gradually adding 1 to 2 cups (1/4 to 1/2 liter) of vegetable oil to the daily ration. When there is not only the question of a degree of malfunction but also very poorly functioning molars, the concentrates can be soaked in warm water. Mash and soaked beet pulp can be consumed with hardly any need to grind. Grass pellets and alfalfa (Lucerne) pellets can also be soaked before being given. At this stage, attention must be paid to the

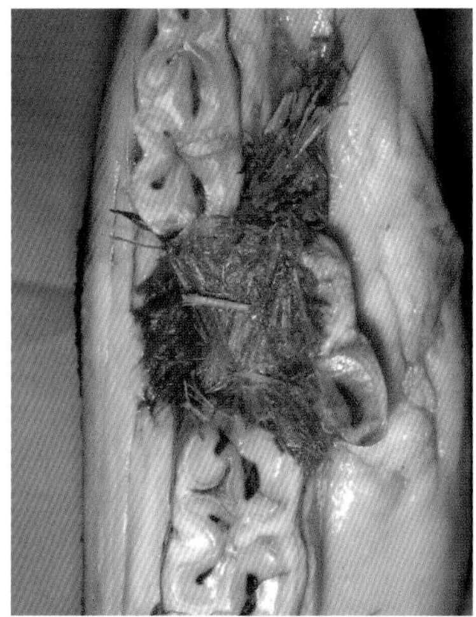

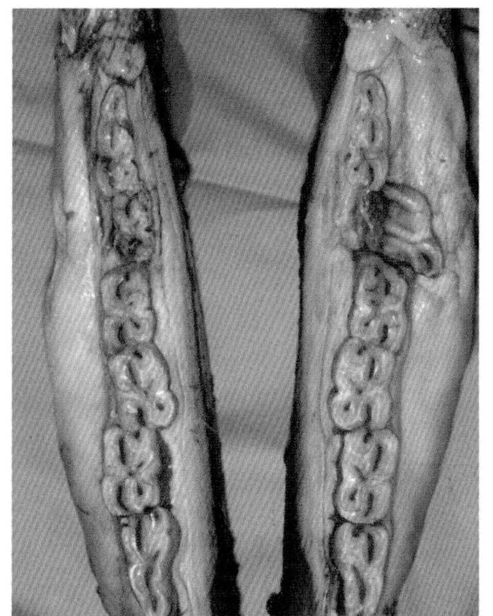

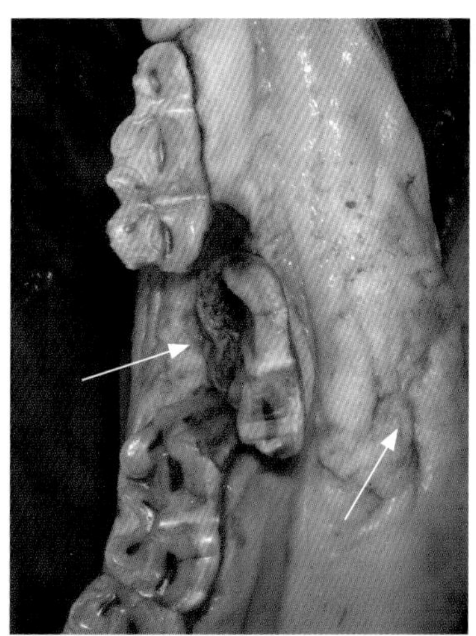

The set of teeth of this older horse shows that it had suffered a lot. A molar had been pushed outward because the inside half had broken off a long time before. This had caused food to be accumulated and had lead to extensive periodontitis. Note also the scars on the soft tissue of the cheek caused by the molar pressing continually into it.

proper balance of vitamins and minerals. Indeed, this type of diet is very different from the normal horse diet.

These days, there are a number of feed products that offer a composition of concentrates specifically designed for the older horse. Some products even have a feed for older horses that is so balanced that any other kind of food is unnecessary.

When, out of sheer necessity, your horse's diet must be changed because of a poorly functioning set of teeth, it is best to consult a veterinarian or an equine diet specialist beforehand.

The dental care of older horses is no longer aimed at the restoration of a normal molar table but at allowing the most comfortable and most efficient possible intake of food. The reducing to "normal" height of a number of teeth that are too long can mean that, in these horses, the grinding table no longer meets the opposite molar which, in turn, means that your horse can barely chew anymore. Theoretically, the molars would then be "correctly" positioned in the mouth but actually, the horse still has difficulty in chewing its food.

Ponies can grow extremely old. I even knew one pony that reached 52 years old. The owner's father gave it to him as a wedding present when it was a yearling; when the owner had his golden wedding anniversary, this pony was still happily trotting along in the wedding party parade!

This 21-year-old Warmblood was brought in—all skin and bone—for euthanasia because, according to its owner, it was "finished." An autopsy quickly revealed why this horse had been so thin.

A. The side view of both lower molar arcades looked rather like a mountain range instead of a level plateau. The gums round both of the first molars in the lower jaw had been completely bitten away by the first upper molar.
B. The side of the tongue was injured by the sharp inside of a lower molar.
C. The inside of the cheek and the gums next to the third lower molar were badly injured by the long enamel points of the upper molars.
D. There were profound accumulations of food in diastemas between various molars.
E. A sharp back hook had caused a cut in the hard palate.

The whole gamut of possible dental defects was present in this horse's mouth. Its last year of life must have been one of great suffering. Regular dental checks and treatment could have prevented all this.

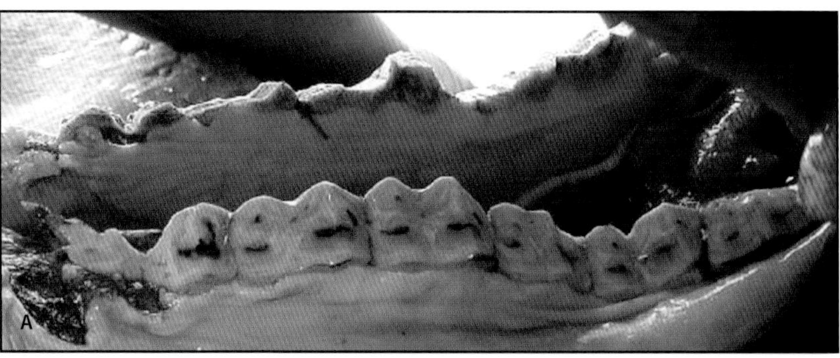
A

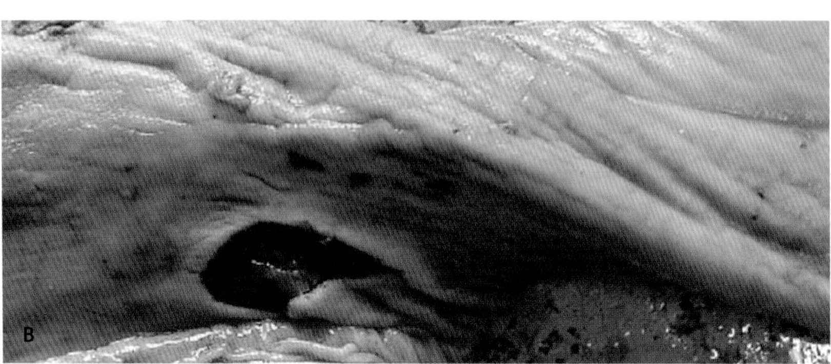
B

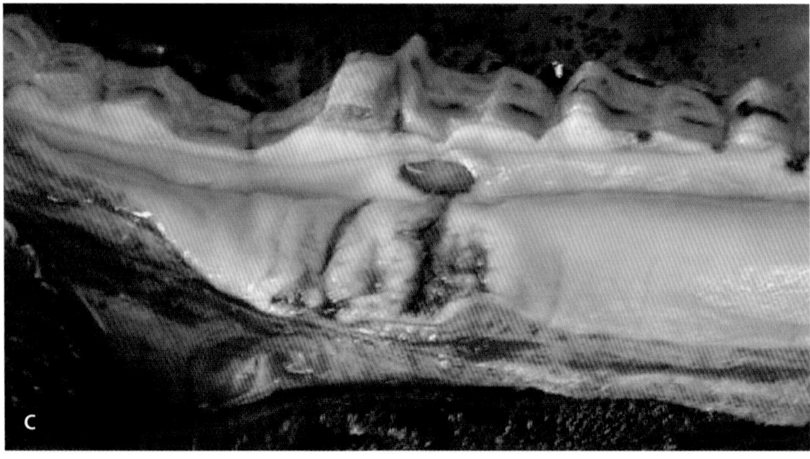
C

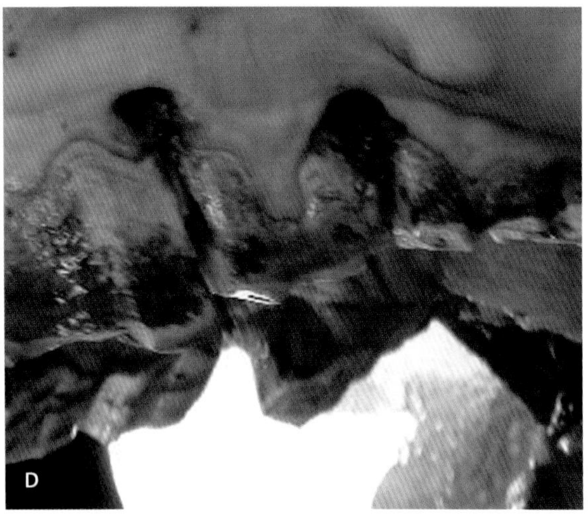
D

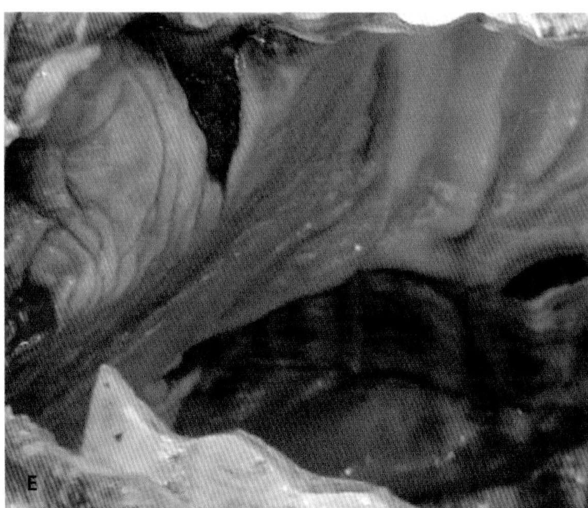
E

CHAPTER 19

Points of Interest by Age

Newly Born Foals

- Overbite
- Underbite
- Congenital defects of the lips or of the palate (cleft)

Six to Nine Months

- Fitting together of the incisors and the first three milk molars
- Missing teeth
- Sharp enamel points or hooks

16 to 24 Months

- Wolf teeth
- Sharp enamel points or hooks
- Injuries caused by the bit on the bars and the corners of the mouth

Two to Three Years

- Late emergence of wolf teeth or blind wolf teeth
- Persistent milk teeth on the incisors and the first three molars
- Injuries caused by the bit
- Wolf teeth

Three to Four Years

- Injuries caused by the bit
- Persistent milk incisors
- Persistent caps on the third molar (.08)
- Sharp enamel points and hooks
- Blind wolf teeth

Five Years and Older

- Injuries caused by the bit
- Sharp enamel points and hooks
- Irregular abrasion of the incisors and molars

The Older Horse

- Hooks and irregular abrasion of the molars
- Irregular abrasion of the incisors
- Plaque round the canines
- Diastemas and periodontitis
- Loose teeth

Glossary

Back hook: A sharp protrusion at the back of the table of the last upper or lower molar.

Bit seats: These are installed by rolling and smoothing the front of the first upper and lower premolars (.06).

Biting plate: A metal plate that is fixed to a bit that protrudes between the incisors. It is used to correct an overbite in foals.

Brachydont: Teeth with a short crown in relation to the root.

Canine: A tooth between the incisors and molars found in male animals. It is sometimes found in a smaller version in female animals.

Caps: The remains of the milk teeth that come loose at the eruption of the permanent teeth. They usually take the form of flat, rectangular-shaped slivers.

Caries (cavities): Damage to the tooth due to bacterial fermentation of sugars in the mouth.

Cementum: The substance that is on the outside of the tooth and in the mark (the enamel cup).

Cheek lesion: An injury on the inside of the cheek.

Dental star: A stain on the nipping surface of the incisors that is caused by the top of the root canal being filled in with dentine as the teeth wear with age.

Dentine: A soft substance that is part of the tooth. As the horse ages, dentine fills up the top of the root canal.

Diastema: An acquired split-like gap between two incisors or two molars.

Dorsal curvature: The lower incisors form a bulge upward into the upper incisors.

Echancrure or notch: The development of a hook at the back of the nipping edge of the upper corner incisors (.03).

Erratic or ectopic teeth: Teeth situated outside the skull that are found just in front of the base of the ear.

Eruption: The breaking through of a tooth into the mouth. It also describes the subsequent emergence of the reserve crown coming out of the socket as the horse ages.

Extraction: The pulling out of a tooth.

Fistula: A suppurating wound emanating from the infected root of a molar.

Floating: Using a dental rasp known as a "float."

Foremost hook: A sharp lengthening of the front part of the table of the first upper or lower molar.

Fulcrum: The apparatus that forms the fulcrum for the extraction forceps. The leverage action of the fulcrum makes it easier to pull a molar.

Enamel: The hardest component of the teeth and, actually, of the whole body.

Enamel cup or mark: A hollow that is formed by an enamel ring that is completely or partly filled with cementum. There is one partly filled enamel cup in the table of the incisors and there are two filled enamel cups situated centrally in the table of the upper molars.

Enamel points: Sharp points of enamel on the outer edge of the tables of the upper molars and on the inner edge of the lower molars. Enamel points are frequently the cause of injury to the soft tissue inside the cheeks.

Enamel "rings": Two indentations centrally situated on the tables of the upper molars.

Galvayne's groove: A groove on the lip side of upper corner incisors (103 and 203). In the past, these were used—incorrectly—to determine the age of a horse.

Gelding tooth: See Canine.

Incisor arc: The arc formed by the nipping surface of all the incisors.

Hook: The table of a molar lies slightly beyond the table of the opposing molar thus a part of the table is no longer worn down and a pointed elevation (hook) develops.

Hypsodont: A high-crowned tooth with a lot of reserve crown, which continually erupts from the socket of the tooth during the life of the horse.

Mandible: The bony part of the skull that forms the lower jaw.

Mandibular bump: A bump on the under side of the lower jaw. It is caused by the replacement of the second or third lower molars.

"Mark": See Enamel cup.

Maxillary: The bony part of the skull that forms the upper jaw.

Maxillary sinuses: The horse's forehead cavities situated just above the roots of the third to the sixth upper molars.

Occlusal surface: The grinding surface that is formed by the two full arcades of molars.

Offset incisors: A defective condition of the contact surface whereby on one side of the mouth the upper incisors are too long and the lower incisors are too short. On the other side of the mouth, the defect is seen in the reverse.

Overbite: The incisors of the upper jaw protrude further forward than the incisors of the lower jaw.

Parotid gland: The biggest salivary gland of the horse situated at the base of the ear and behind the jaw.

Periodontitis: An inflammation of the tissue (gums) outside and around the tooth.

Persistent caps: The last part of a milk tooth that remains in the mouth for too long.

Persistent milk incisor: A milk incisor that remains in the mouth for too long.

"Punching out" (trephining of teeth): The extraction of a molar through an opening to the outside of the skull using a hammer and trephine punch.

Quidding: The act of dropping partially chewed food from the mouth. (See Wads or balls.)

Ramps: The whole table of a molar slants upward toward one end. This is usually seen in the first or the last molars of the lower jaw.

Reserve crown: The part of the crown under the gums that is situated in the socket.

Root canal: The canal through which blood vessels and nerves pass from the root cavity to the crown of the tooth.

Root cavity: A space inside the root of the tooth where blood vessels and nerves are found.

Root elevator: A hand instrument designed to work the root of a tooth free from the socket.

Sedative: A drug that anesthetizes somewhat. It mainly has a calming effect and at the same time it is a mild painkiller.

Shear mouth: The slope (angle) of the tables of opposing molars is far too oblique; a sideways movement of the jaws is practically impossible.

Sinuses: Sinus cavities.

Sinusitis: An infection of the sinus cavity.

Socket: Bony structures which hold the teeth in place.

Soft teeth: Teeth where the crown is already worn down to just above the root. The hard tooth enamel is no longer present on the table.

Spee curvature: The upward curving of the last lower molars.

Squirreling: The act of hoarding food between the cheeks and outer side of the molars that usually indicates a serious dental defect.

Stallion tooth: See Canine.

Step incisor: An incisor with a taller table as compared to the neighbouring incisors.

Step mouth: A condition where the table of a tooth is obviously taller than the tables of surrounding teeth.

Tooth bud: An embryonic rudimentary form of a tooth.

Transverse ridges: Crosswise protrusions at right angles to the linear direction of the arcade of molars. There are 11 to 13 transverse ridges to each arcade.

Trephine punch: A blunt metal chisel used to extract molars from the outside of the head.

Trephining: See "Punching out."

Triadan numbering: The numbering developed by Triadan to identify each specific tooth in the mouth.

Underbite: The incisors of the lower jaw protrude further forward than the incisors of the upper jaw.

Ventral curvature: The upper incisors form a bulge downward into the lower incisors.

Visible crown: The part of the crown of the tooth that rises above the gums in the mouth.

Wads or balls: Partly chewed hay or grass the horse lets drop from its mouth, an act known as "quidding."

Wave mouth: Upward or downward curving of the arcades of molars involving several teeth.

Wolf tooth: A small tooth just in front of the first upper molars. Very occasionally found in front of the lower molars.

Index

Page numbers in *italic* indicate photographs or illustrations.